Headscape

Headscape

*How a bald guy replanted his hair
and restarted his life*

Chris Schroder
January 24, 2023

Chris Schroder

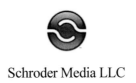

Schroder Media LLC

ISBN: 979-8-9861676-3-3 (Paperback)

Library of Congress Control Number: 2022907622

This book is a personal memoir based on the memories of the author. Some names have been omitted or reduced to first names to protect the identities of those involved.

Cover design by Heidi Rizzi, Pixel Perfect Design
Book design by Chris Schroder
Edited by Jan Schroder and James "Tripp" Griffin
Printed by BookLogix, in the United States of America

First printing edition, May 2022.

Schroder Media LLC
P.O. Box 250026
Atlanta, GA 30325

www.schrodermedia.com
www.headscape.me

Dedicated to my wife Jan,
who humors my countless creative ideas,
judiciously edits my work
and continuously blesses my life.

"The hoary head is a crown of glory,
if it be found in the way of righteousness."

– Proverbs 16:31

Contents

Preface

For years, when I'd talk with people in person, I'd notice their gaze drifting up toward my bald head. I'd always wonder what it was they were noticing: my shiny skin, the one or two remaining hairs randomly growing on an otherwise barren landscape or perhaps the minor scars where I'd hit my head on a door frame.

Today, the same thing happens, and I still wonder what they are thinking – yet I am no longer bald.

Chris Schroder
Lake James, North Carolina
May 2022

1. My First Haircut

L ike my two children, I was born bald, only to grow in a few hairs as I approached six months of age. It grew slowly, finally stepping up its pace by the time of my first trip to an official barber shop run by Mr. Evans, a kindly older gentleman with little hair himself who ran a traditional tonsorium located in Rhodes Center, a 1930s-era marble-clad strip of stores adjacent to the 1904 historical mansion, Rhodes Hall, in Midtown Atlanta's Ansley Park. My mother and siblings had been making a big deal in the days leading up to my first haircut and joining in the family tradition of visiting Mr. Evans.

On the appointed day, a hot, muggy weekday afternoon, my brothers and I were already sweating as we walked the two blocks from our family's home in the Palace Apartments at Spring and Peachtree streets. On the outside wall, there was the traditional red-and-blue-and-white turning barber's pole, which thankfully I didn't know then dates back hundreds of years to barbers' origins as hair-trimmers and blood-letters. I was already terrified enough of this thing called a haircut. Above the glass door there was a large, loud air conditioning unit that dripped water onto the hot pavement. On the windows were large letters with the name of the shop and even larger letters spelling out "Now with Air-Conditioning."

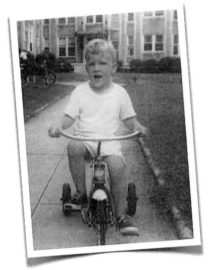 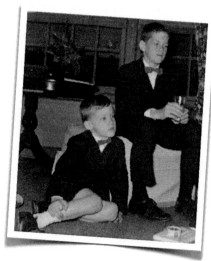

**Almost 3: At Atlanta's Palace Apartments,
before my first haircut at Mr. Evans' Rhodes Center shop.
Age 5: After several haircuts, with brother Mike.**

When we opened the door, I was amazed by the change in environment. The air conditioning blasted us with frigid air and the room was deafeningly loud with men's voices and laughter. On the left side of the shop were two chairs and Mr. Evans, wearing a starched white shirt, light gray jacket, and small round spectacles. He was busy cutting the hair of one customer.

"Come in gentlemen," he said as we entered. We stood by the windows as the chairs against the right and back walls of the shop were full of middle-aged men, all dressed in dark suits and ties with large leather briefcases resting next to their dark shoes. I was a shy child and all this noise scared me. Mr. Evans seemed nice though and he recognized my fear. When his customer stepped out of the chair, he put up a wooden shelf across the arms of the big

2

leather-and-metal chair. A Black man walked from the back of the shop with a small broom and swept the previous customer's hair on the floor and chair into an old metal dustpan and then retreated to the back room.

"Step up, young man," Mr. Evans said to me.

"What about your other customers who were here first?" one of my brothers asked, pointing to the crowd of men in the chairs.

"Oh, they're just salesmen stealing my air conditioning," Mr. Evans said. "Don't mind them. They don't need haircuts."

As I sat on the wooden shelf, Mr. Evans tied a striped sheet around my neck and draped it over my legs and the chair. He grabbed an old silver metal razor and brought it close to me and turned it on. The loud sound scared me and I wiggled to try to escape the chair. My brothers smiled. All the men in the room started laughing. Mr. Evans told them to quiet down and he turned off the razor, nudged me back in the chair, and grabbed scissors and a black comb and started carefully trimming the edges of my uneven head of hair. It felt good as he gently patted my head and stroked it with his comb. I didn't mind the scissor sound as they clipped, dropping strands of my hair to the floor for the Black gentleman to sweep up later.

As I sat there, I listened to the men in the chairs. One was telling a story of a woman he knew who had been found dead in her apartment.

"The police came and they couldn't figure out how she died," he said. "They determined the last thing she ate was chocolate-covered graham crackers. She had several packs in her freezer and they decided she must have had a bad reaction to the chocolate-covered graham crackers and died."

I looked at my brothers in fear. We had a pack of chocolate-covered graham crackers in our freezer in our apartment. I had eaten many of them and had liked them, but after I stepped down from Mr. Evans' chair, I told my brothers I was never going to eat them again.

To this day, I haven't eaten any – and this event may have impacted the fact I don't really enjoy the campfire tradition of s'mores, a combination of graham crackers, Hershey's chocolate, and marshmallows. I've never cared much since for haircuts or barber shops either.

2. My Best Hair Day Ever

T he best hair day of my life was in seventh grade when the yearbook photographer took a photo of our class officers. My hair looked near-perfect that day – full, clinging smartly across my head with a slight curl down and across my forehead. Back then, I thought I would have that head of hair all my life, even if it one day turned gray. I was proud of my hair, thinking it was one of my most appealing attributes.

A year later, when the annual published our eighth-grade officer photos, my look had changed slightly: I had begun nurturing a creeping widow's peak. I much preferred my seventh-grade photo, yet my destiny was writ atop my forehead for all to see.

There were many years when I blamed myself for the loss of my hair on an unhealthy habit I began in seventh grade. I had just transferred from my parochial grade school to a larger, more challenging independent school. There was a lot more homework. My family had also just moved to a new house and my bedroom had a small desk built into the chimney shaft.

I had never been a focused reader or student. I have a creative mind and it wanders at will, particularly when I read long texts. Perhaps as a nervous habit, I started rubbing and scratching my scalp, perhaps being comforted by the tiny detritus that fell on the

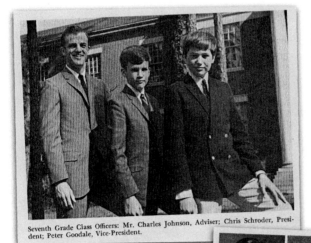

Age 12: My best hair day ever was in seventh grade.

(I was actually class vice president).

Seventh Grade Class Officers: Mr. Charles Johnson, Adviser; Chris Schroder, President; Peter Goodale, Vice-President.

Age 13: The dreaded widow's peak makes its first appearance in eighth grade.

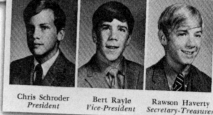

Chris Schroder
President

Bert Rayle
Vice-President

Rawson Haverty
Secretary-Treasurer

desk. As I sat there for hours each school night, the scratching and removal of the top layer of skin around my follicles went on without me even noticing. I don't remember seeing any hair fall out – I'd hoped I wasn't digging into the follicle roots – nevertheless, I was certainly altering the terrain and probably not for the better.

At the time, a frequent Head n' Shoulders shampoo TV commercial lifted the word dandruff to a terrifying syndrome. In it a man on a date was wearing a dark coat and the very moment the woman touched his shoulder in a presumed lean-in for a kiss, she looked down and saw – horrors – dandruff on his shoulder, brushed it off, and recoiled from the cuddle. A part of me thought I might be removing dandruff, which I certainly did not want to fall on my shoulders at school. What would the girls in my class think?

As my hair began to shrink its shape following my best-hair days, I cultivated a growing sense of shame that I might have been the cause of my hair's own demise. As the widow's peak began to grow, my mother was concerned I'd soon resemble her bald father-in-law, my paternal grandfather whom I never met. She took me to her dermatologist for early intervention when I was in high school.

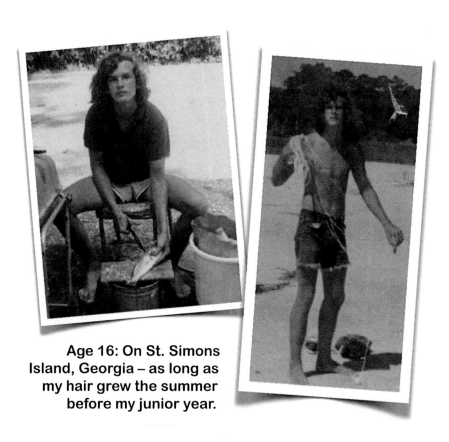

Age 16: On St. Simons Island, Georgia – as long as my hair grew the summer before my junior year.

"There's nothing we can do," he diagnosed. "This is classic male pattern baldness. It's genetic. Just get used to it. He's going bald."

As we began to leave his office, I quietly told the doctor of my nervous junior-high study habit and asked if I might have brought on what he called male pattern baldness.

"I don't believe so," he said after further studying the pores on my head with a magnifying glass. "These areas don't show damage, they just show a symmetrical pattern of loss as the hair follicle root dies, the hair shaft falls out, and the skin joins its hairless neighbors. I don't think you need to blame yourself. This is a genetic situation."

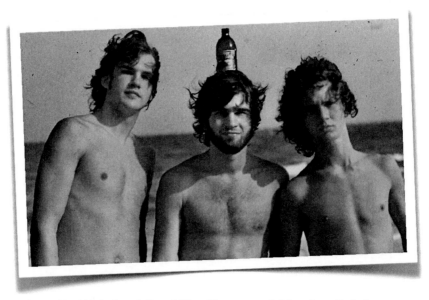

Age 17: With buddies Mike Egan and Charles Driebe on Tybee Island, Georgia in a memorable photo we reprinted for decades on birthday invitations, though Mike requested we remove the beer bottle during his storied legal career.

There was some small comfort, given his sad prognosis, that I didn't have to blame myself for my baldness that was looming above me much like an old-fashioned summer thunderstorm from the west. I could now just blame my ancestors.

My hair reached its longest length when I was 16, my junior year in high school, right when I returned to Westminster after more than two years at boarding school at Georgetown Prep. The long curls and waves wandered down to my shoulder blades. Then, as college approached and styles changed, I began to clip it shorter, just over my collar. The thick hair on the sides and in the back offset the prominent forehead – at least in my mind.

Will we ever have another bald president?

Dwight Eisenhower was our last elected bald president. Some question his eligibility as he sometimes shaved his head. Also, he twice defeated Adlai Stevenson II, who may have had less hair than Ike.

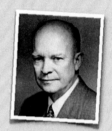

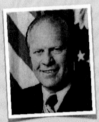

Gerald Ford was technically our last bald president, but if we are discussing whether another bald guy could ever be elected president … Ford was never actually elected.

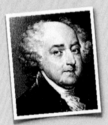 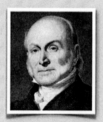 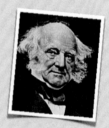

Otherwise you may have to go back to pre-1850 and **John Adams, John Quincy Adams** and **Martin Van Buren.**

John Delaney was the first candidate to enter the 2020 Democratic primary. Sharp guy, but never polled 2%.

Joe Biden was elected 33 years after telling a reporter, hot on his hair transplant story, "Guess. I've got to keep some mystery."

3. The End of the Comb-over

During my first wedding at age 22 – three weeks after the partial meltdown of nuclear reactor number 2 on Pennsylvania's Three Mile Island – college fraternity brother Hank West grabbed the small remaining dollop of my brown forehead hair, proclaiming to the entire wedding party, "Two Mile Island!" Karma descended upon Hank as he became a Charleston, South Carolina surgeon, eventually becoming leader of the state medical society. His long, sandy brown hair receded dramatically and his baldness caught up and had exceeded my own.

For the next decade, as an itinerant newspaperman, I dragged my wife, her golden retriever Hephzibah, and a feral cat we found in Greenville, Mississippi and named Greenwich from state to state for the allure of $30-a-week increase in salary. Along the way, I charted my own follicle fallout.

When my new bride brought a few antiques to my Mississippi Delta garage apartment, I realized it was time to invest in something mature: renters' insurance. So I called around town, secured the best price and then drove my wife to the insurance firm to sign our policy. The secretary asked us to wait in the lobby and she called the middle-aged insurance agent to come up front to

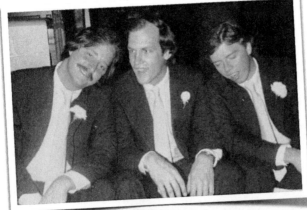

Age 22: "Two Mile Island" appears above with Irénée May, left, and Norris Broyles, right, at my first wedding.

Age 22: Interviewing presidential candidate George H.W. Bush at the Augusta, Georgia, airport.

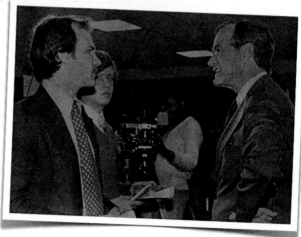

meet us. He walked out of the back office wearing the local business uniform: a sleeveless white T-Shirt under a short-sleeved, white collared business shirt and a short striped tie. He adjusted his glasses, stuck his hand out and said, "Hello, Mr. Schroder. Welcome." After we shook hands, he looked to his right and briefly studied my wife.

"And this," he said in his best Delta drawl, "This must be your lovely daughter."

Had I not been in a hurry – and had he not already qualified himself with the cheapest policy in town – I might have taken our small check elsewhere. I realized my wife, six months my junior, looked young, but I rationalized his embarrassing remark with the thought I must have looked very mature that day.

On the third stop of our Southern tour, Greenville, South Carolina, I caught the eye of the young cavalier publisher, Bern Mebane. A North Carolina grad with slightly more hair than me, he had a penchant for promoting his managers and then assigning and deploying patronizing nicknames. Whenever I entered his orbit the next three years, he'd proclaim – "Herr Schroder!" – prompting his reports to grin on cue as he cleverly mocked my German last name and, it seemed, my departing hair.

I learned to cope well enough with my growing pate as our daughter and son grew into toddlers. I discovered if I parted my hair a bit lower on my parietal ridge, I could cajole enough follicles from the ample mélange above my left temple to wander surreptitiously over my vertex, eventually weaving into the hodgepodge on my right temple. This comb-over worked fine, probably fooling no one, especially when I jumped in a pool or if a sudden breeze blew across.

Following a later move from Charlotte back to our hometown of Atlanta, I decided I needed a weekend in the woods, setting my sights on the highest mountaintop east of the Rockies, Mt. Mitchell, North Carolina. On my first full day, I set off on a long downhill hike through Eraser's Fir trees that nearly covered the rocky, clay path. The archway apex provided just enough gap that while I wandered the dense forest, I was warmed by the sun that lit my path. All seemed great until I awoke the next morning in my tent with what I first thought was a blazing headache.

When I reached up, touched my head, and squelched, I discovered my scalp below my thin covering of hair had overnight morphed into a Mars-like landscape of singed red skin. I rummaged through my car trunk, finding the cap that I wished I'd remembered the day before. Pulling that on proved painful. I started down another path and screamed in pain when I didn't stoop low enough under a tree limb, driving the metal cap button into my inflamed skin. I turned around and broke camp.

Driving back to Atlanta, I rotated through my three favorite road trip cassettes: Ten Years After's *A Space in Time*, The Who's *Who's Next*, followed by Crosby, Stills, Nash & Young's *Déjà Vu*. As David Crosby sang "letting my freak flag fly" on "Almost Cut

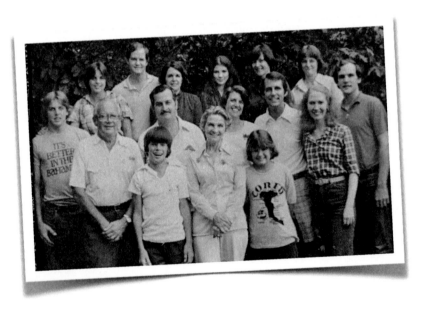

Age 22: Most everyone in my family had more hair than me.

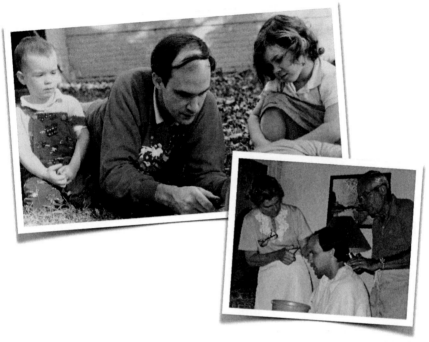

**Age 29: Attempting a comb-over while carving a pumpkin in
Charlotte with son, Thomas and daughter, Sally;
my mom and dad giving me a haircut.**

My Hair," the album's third track, I concluded my days of flying
my own freak flag had flown by.

I drove straight to my barber. "Cut it," I said. "I'm 33 and I'm
not hiding it anymore. Do be careful, I'm badly sunburned."

I drove home wearing my cap and unveiled it at the dinner table.
My kids giggled. My wife gasped a bit. "This is the new me," I
said. "Such as it is."

When I walked through the advertising department of the *Atlanta
Journal-Constitution* the next morning, where I had recently been
hired as Creative Director, I took notice of all the salespeople's

double-takes. I walked into the art department, greeted my design team and, as they began to look up and stare, I walked into my office. Joey, a talented artist who was gay, knocked on my door.

"You got quite a haircut!" he said, smiling. I grimaced and shrugged my shoulders.

"I figured it was time to stop hiding it," I said.

"I like bald guys," he said. "It's a good look. But you're lucky."

"Why?" I asked.

"Not all men have good-looking bald heads," he said. "You have a very nice one." I blushed.

My next appearance was in front of my sisters, brothers, and parents. My dad and his maternal grandfather, whom he adored and whose severe portrait loomed over our mantle for as long as I remember, each had receding hairlines, but managed to cultivate a healthy tuft of hair on the center of their foreheads that they brushed straight back. My oldest brother Jack, eight years older, to this day cultivates a head full of thick dark hair. My next brother Mike, six years my senior, introduced our family to the hippie look when he arrived home early from college in 1970 after students rioted and shut down campuses nationwide. While still nicely coiffed, he was thinning a bit, though not noticeably – yet.

I felt cheated, having older brothers and a dad with more hair than me. "I'm looking forward to growing older," I told them. "In our family, apparently, the older you get, the more hair you grow. I look forward to catching up one day."

My mom, as always, made the best of it. "Your father's father was bald and very handsome – and you are too," she said. "But I'm really proud of you. I can't stand it when men do those comb-overs on TV. When I see those news anchors doing that or wearing toupees, I just want to reach into that TV and snatch it right off their heads!"

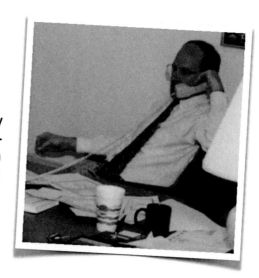

Age 35: In my Atlanta Journal-Constitution office – the final weeks of my sporting the dreaded comb-over.

Despite everyone's encouragement, I wasn't comfortable with my new look. I invested in nice English driving caps, baseball caps and even a fedora. Fearing I'd burn my scalp, I rarely ever again went outside without wearing a cap.

I soon realized I had no further use for a comb and I didn't really have to brush my hair anymore, even after a shower. I just ran my hands down the sides of my head and I was good to go. I cultivated a new excuse whenever I was late: "Sorry, I had to do my hair."

From my perspective, the world seemed the same – yet I wasn't. When people's eyes drifted above my gaze, I wondered if my bald skin moved when I talked or if I'd sprouted freckles or pimples.

"I'm just being self-conscious," I'd counsel myself, until I'd walk by a mirror or glass storefront. Then, I'd be shocked by my image reflected back. I didn't recognize that me. I might feel the same and the voice coming from within sounded the same, but that person in the mirror – that guy with the bright white dome – that wasn't the me I knew. Where did *that* guy go?

4. When A Lot More Than My Hair Fell Out

Soon enough, I began to wonder where our marriage was going. The stress of moving from town to town was apparently taking its toll on my wife. She was a deep introvert and had few close friends. In Greenville, South Carolina, she had become close to a young mother who lived up the street from us. As we were packing up our house to move to my next job at *The Charlotte Observer*, the neighbor pulled me aside and spoke quietly.

"This move will not be good for your wife," she warned. "It would be better for her if you stayed here. I know what I'm talking about." Her words scared me, but I dismissed her warning, saying my wife and I compared ourselves to bonsai plants, lifting ourselves up, clipping our roots and settling in a new pot up the road with maturing, though perhaps clipped branches.

Nearly five years later, on our final move as a couple, my wife and I purchased a gorgeous 1904 Tudor home near the entrance of Ansley Park in the shadow of Midtown Atlanta's skyscrapers – less than 150 yards from the now-empty shell of Mr. Evans' old barber shop. I had taken a job with the *Atlanta Journal-Constitution* which I had read every morning at the breakfast table with my father. I had always dreamed of returning the paper to its early glory. My buddy Charles Driebe, who had been my business partner for four summers in college in a bricklaying company and had since trailed me in our own personal race to baldness, seemed envious. "Dude," he said. "You are at the center of the universe."

The truth was, my wife and I had always been house-poor. We invested every extra cent we had in buying, renovating, and selling older intown homes in our perpetual game of hopscotch. On my newspaper salary, we couldn't afford to dine at nice restaurants with friends or take luxury vacations, but we had comforted ourselves that we lived in nice older homes around the South. While we felt fortunate to buy this historic home during a recession for less than $300,000, it was not financially viable for us.

With my wife staying home to raise children and me earning $52,000 at the daily paper – even with our sizable downpayment netted from the sale of the 1929 Craftsman home on Charlotte's Dilworth Road West that we had renovated – it wasn't smart. This beautiful home was not our normal fixer-upper. We had to renovate every surface – cove ceilings, hardwood floors, plaster walls – and we couldn't afford to live anywhere other than amidst the constant dust and disorder with our two children, our dog, a cat, and a hamster.

We began to fight more often and intensely. We had painted our front living room a gorgeous Victorian shade of rich, dark red. When my father-in-law walked in and saw the color for the first time, he looked around and growled, "This color makes me want to fight!" It was the oddest of statements, but perhaps a familial telling one.

Despite losing my youthful locks, I was determined to re-enter my hometown with panache. We mailed a change-of-address announcement that began, "After 12 long years, 11 anniversaries,

10 moving vans, 9 hundred miles, 8 promotions, 7 addresses, 6 newspapers, 5 cars, 4 towns, 3 dogs, 2 cats and 1 huge sigh of relief …"

I recruited buddies who'd also just returned to Atlanta from more exotic locales such as Germany, New York, and London to throw a joint "The Boys are Back in Town" party, offering our house as the venue. My wife agreed but was not happy about it. We both worked on the house every spare moment we had in the weeks leading up to the event. We fought over falling wallpaper, wobbly slate floors, and new kitchen cabinets. Finally, with our house

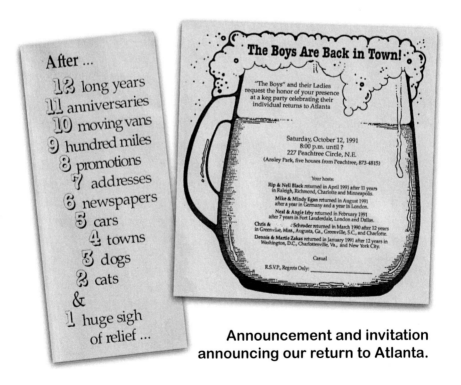

Announcement and invitation announcing our return to Atlanta.

filled with guests I was so eager to impress, I looked across the red living room at my wife, noticing for the first time her look of exhaustion etched in the dark semi-circles under her eyes.

A few days later, a classmate she hadn't seen since college jogged past our house. They struck up a conversation at the neighborhood grocery and rekindled their friendship. Another college boyfriend started going to movies with her on Sunday afternoons. I trusted her new relationships were platonic and I surmised that, after moving, raising two children, and putting up with me, she deserved some grace. One thing I did notice: her new friends all had full heads of hair, one flowing down beyond his shoulders.

Had I been more emotionally mature, self-aware, and less exhausted myself, I perhaps would not have grown increasingly uneasy with these sudden challengers who appeared alongside our relationship. Instead, I perhaps should have leaned in, been more sensitive, and paid closer attention to her deepening emotional crevasse.

By one measure, I knew I could not compete with her new interests: I was not capable, no matter how much I wished, of growing more hair. It may seem fatuous in retrospect, but inside my own messy web of insecurities, unhappiness, and rage that had begun to rival my wife's, I seethed with jealousy. Instead of turning to each other, we fought more, pushed each other away, and eventually yanked the ripcord and separated.

A week later – at the newspaper that since childhood I'd told nearly everyone I wanted one day to lead – my new boss fired me. A week after that, I was rushed to the hospital for emergency appendix surgery, followed by a staph infection that extended my hospitalization for a week. I had never spent a night in a hospital before. As I recovered in my hospital room after a tumultuous four weeks in April, I took inventory of my life. I wasn't happy with my summation.

Since I was without work that summer, drawing $235 a week unemployment, my wife found a job in a school development office. Our relationship grew more confused as she sprouted new wings. Three months later, my children informed me their mother was seeing a new guy, a friend of someone at her school. This being before Facebook or Google, I had no idea who he was or what he looked like, but I certainly had my fears.

A few weeks later, her brilliant uncle, a former congressman, distinguished jurist and state supreme court justice, died of cancer. I noted the scheduling of his memorial service at the state justice building a block from a daily legal newspaper where I'd finally been offered a job in late August. I wasn't invited to the service and I feared my soon-to-be ex-wife and her new interest (and soon enough new husband) would be there. I asked a legal reporter covering the event to act as my spy. When she returned, the journalist glibly delivered her report.

"Your wife was there, introducing who appeared to be her new guy all around the room," she said.

The dagger was not in far enough apparently – I had to ask. "What does he look like?"

"Just a suit," she said, adding before walking back to her computer, "but he does have great hair."

DILBERT SCOTT ADAMS

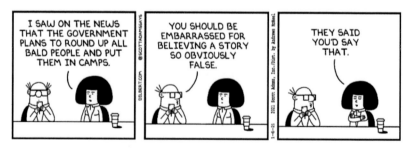

5. The Summer of My German Tutor

I left the next day with my children, my parents, and my brother Mike for a long-planned week's vacation at a St. Simons Island, Georgia rental home. I had agreed to rendezvous with my wife three days later in Macon so she could take our children to her uncle's funeral.

At 9:30 a.m. on my first weekday morning at the coast, my wife called with news: she had changed her mind about waiting a few months to file our provisionally signed divorce papers and had filed them that morning at the Fulton County Courthouse. With a judge's signature in 30 days, our marriage would be dissolved.

Sally and Thomas were asleep in the next room. Shaken, I went to the kitchen and saw Mike. Our family was not one to share emotions – particularly bad ones. I began fixing a large cooler of gin and tonics. I told Mike of my call with my wife and my sudden need to go to the beach and begin drinking heavily, asking if he'd keep an eye on my kids when they awakened. I donned a baseball cap, grabbed my cooler and headed out, tears streaming.

I wanted to be miles away from everyone. I walked to an isolated patch of sand on the elbow at East Beach, spread out my towel, and covered the cooler to shade my medicine from the hot Georgia sun. I began assessing the damage as, clearly, my wife had moved on. I inventoried my assets: I was an almost-divorced dad with a college degree, zero cash in the bank, living on unemployment with a new obligation to pay monthly child support, living again in my parents' basement, co-owner of a house of which I bequeathed the majority to my wife in lieu of alimony and – perhaps most damning of all – bald.

I had felt the pull of this swirl before – that perilous, depressed pity spiral that had drawn me towards its devilish destination. This pit seemed like a bottomless one. Normally, the sun and surf could comfort me, but not today. The humidity seemed heavy on my shoulders and the wind blew stinging waves of sand into my legs.

I looked to my right, noticing for the first time a towel 50 yards away. A book held it in place. Needing solitude, I planned to move further down the beach.

Then, a tall, sinewy woman walked out of the waves, squeezing salt water from her long blonde hair. I watched as she lay face down on her towel, unbuckled her bikini top, grabbed her book, and turned her head the other direction.

Admittedly, I was not thinking clearly.

I wondered if I should ignore her and move. Or was this perhaps a biblical test of my resolve, my faithfulness here as I neared a state-imposed deadline. Was this a test commissioned by God – or worse, a ploy concocted by my wife's attorney to squeeze me for further support? Or was it instead a life preserver thrown by God, to whom I had only that spring begun to cry out for help. Or, less celestially, had the universe suddenly cast me in a beer commercial?

I shook my head. I was no doubt assigning too much gravity to a woman who'd merely tossed her towel nearby before I arrived on that same lonely stretch of coastline. Thirty days, I thought, and I'll be divorced. I should wait. After all, I was in a very fragile state. Rejection now would only hasten my descent.

I proffered the absurdity of it – she was probably too young for me. If I approached her, I might be perceived as a creepy old man. On the other hand, what did I, already a loser, have to lose? I couldn't descend any lower than the sand I was sitting on. If this blonde rejected me, would it really hurt in light of that morning's news? Would I even feel the pain in my shocked state?

Fueled by the gin perhaps, I took the gamble, walked over, and said, "Hello, would you like some company?"

She turned, re-fastened her top, leaned up on her elbows, squinted in the bright sun and said matter-of-factly: "Ja."

I quickly grabbed my items, spread my towel and cooler next to her. After a moment, I asked her, "Would you like a gin and tonic?"

"It is early, ja?" she said.

"Well," I stuttered, "yes, but I've already had a bad day. Are you … German … or Swedish?"

"Ja, my name is Maria. I'm from Berlin. I have never been out of my country before," she said in an elegant, slightly severe English. "My uncle invited me for the summer to teach his children German. This is my morning off."

She was quiet for a moment, looking down the beach. "I have not met anyone on this island close to my age."

I poured her a gin and tonic. She smiled, taking it.

"I am sorry," she said.

"Sorry for what?" I asked.

"I understand Americans are very buttoned up … how do you say … prudish. I prefer sunbathing without a top and I found this beach, where I could swim and sunbathe alone. I didn't realize you were here. I'm sorry if I intruded. I am perhaps, how do you say, a free-spirited person."

"You do not have to apologize, I'm the intruder," I said. "I think you should be as free as you like. Though I should apologize. I'm not really your age. I'm 35."

"It does not matter," she said. "I am 22. We can be friends, no?"

I decided it was time. I took off my cap. "And I'm bald."

She giggled. "It does not matter to me," she said. A few minutes of silence passed. "I'm not like Americans," she said. "I like to jog barefooted. I am going for a run soon. Would you like to run with me?"

"Sure," I said, feigning hesitation. I put on my socks and started putting on my running shoes.

"You should try running barefoot. I believe you will like it," she said.

We left our towels, our shoes, her book, and my cooler as we ran south toward the Coast Guard station and its more crowded public beach. As we passed the entrance, I glanced up the parking lot ramp and saw Mike carrying a towel and a beach chair. I waved. He stopped and watched us run by. He looked confused.

When we returned to our towels, Maria said, "I'm sorry but I must go. I have to go teach my niece and nephew this afternoon."

"I understand," I said. "May I ask you to have a drink tonight?" I asked.

"No, I'm so sorry," she said. "My uncle is taking us all to dinner."

That didn't hurt too bad. I was going to be okay with this ending here. I nodded.

She twisted her hair in a bun, slid on a T-shirt and gathered her items. "Would you be able to meet me after dinner?"

I agreed. She gave me her uncle's address. We hugged and departed in different directions. Back at the house, my children were in the den watching TV. My mom was finishing lunch. A few minutes later, Mike walked in.

"Did I see you a little while ago …?" he whispered.

"Yes," I said. "I can't explain anything that's happening right now."

Two days later, I met my wife in Macon to hand off our children. As our son and daughter visited the restrooms, we shared a few awkward moments alone. I was confused. I felt no anger toward her at that moment. We were being more pleasant than we had been in months. I asked if she needed any cash for the drive back. She cocked her head to the side and said, "What's wrong with you? You're acting different. Did you get laid or something?"

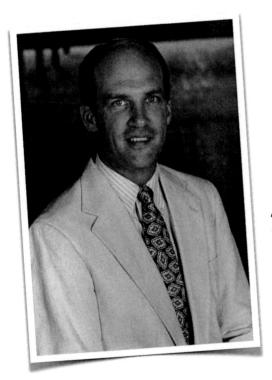

Age 36: On my first day at the Daily Report, following the 30 days in which I lost my job, marriage and appendix – and my summer of divorce, depression, and dalliance.

29

I shook my head, blushed and when my kids returned, hugged them goodbye. They drove north to Atlanta and I returned to the coast for three more days with my family – and with Maria.

Maria's embrace of me at that delicate moment in my life gave me a boost of confidence that lasted for years. We corresponded for a year or two afterwards, but eventually lost touch. I recently tried to contact her on Facebook to thank her for kindness, but if it was her, she didn't respond. Ever since, I've branded that rejuvenating week the "Summer of My German Tutor."

*Quick, name a bald
late night talk show host ...*

... Yeah, that was a hard one.

*Okay, maybe
news anchors or actors?*

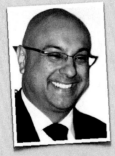

Ali Velshi, who has been an anchor on MSNBC and CNN, said in 2011, "It would be a bald-faced lie to say I haven't enjoyed being king of the follically challenged castle on TV news."

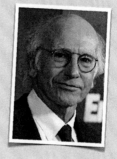

Larry David, accepting the 1992 Emmy for outstanding writing in a comedy series for Seinfeld's "The Contest," told the audience: "This is all very well and good, but I'm still bald."

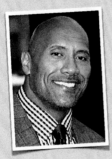

Dwayne "The Rock" Johnson, doesn't have male pattern baldness, but proudly represents the shavers. He tweeted: "I'm bald because my hair is a cross between an afro and hair from a Llama's ball sack."

6. John Malkovich, James Taylor and Coneheads

O ver the next two years, I continued working at the daily legal newspaper and did my best to rebuild resources. Scarred from my previous life of living on a financial razor's edge, I vowed never to go into debt again, except for a mortgage. I also wanted a place of my own so my children wouldn't have to stay overnight at their grandparents' house when I had custody of them three hours on Wednesday nights and every other weekend.

With my fraction of the proceeds from the sale of our marital home, I bought a small house in 1994 for $164,000 in Atlanta's emerging Virginia-Highland/Morningside neighborhood. My dating life was sporadic as I wasn't able to afford frequent dinners out. When I did venture past a first date with a woman, I began to notice a similar pattern: those who seemed most attracted to me had fathers with little to no hair.

I focused on work, precious time with my children, and visiting and staying with my fraternity brothers and their wives who lived within driving distance in Birmingham and Charleston. I also visited a roommate in New York when business took me there. Flying back from New York in time for Atlanta's hosting of its first Super Bowl in January 1994, I read a book on positive personal reinforcement with motivational essays on pushing yourself to focus on others and reflecting their energy.

It seemed trite, but I decided to give it a try. After returning from the airport, I put on cowboy boots and my best jeans, drove downtown into the Super Bowl crowd, and wandered into a music club on Trinity Avenue to hear a local band named GuruFish, pushing my way into the crowd. I began to focus on a group of two women and one man near the stage who were smiling, laughing, and grooving. Remembering the book, I maneuvered myself closer to them as if I was in their group.

I began talking with one woman as if we were old friends. She later told me she assumed, because I was so naturally friendly with her group, that I knew one of them. When the two women were

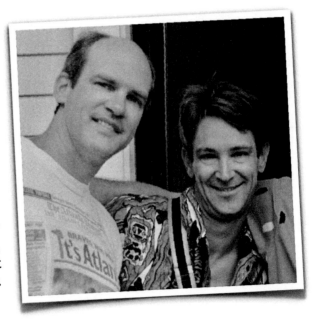

Age 39: In my new single-again years, I often followed high school and college classmate, TC, Dr. Tom Calk to music festivals and concerts. He, like many of my buddies, never lost any of his hair.

ready to leave by taxi, I offered them a ride home, getting the card of the woman in the front seat, an architect named Edith. We began dating the next week. When she invited me to her home for dinner, I looked at photos of her family. Her dad, whom she spoke of reverently, had died a few years prior. I looked carefully at him in group photos. He had less hair than I did.

Once, when looking at older houses along Dearing Street in Athens, Georgia, the sun was behind us and cast our shadows sharply on the sidewalk. I took my cap off, leaned my head back slightly and pointed out to her that the angled shadow of my promontory formed a perfect silhouette of one of *Saturday Night Live*'s Coneheads characters. When she looked on the sidewalk, she nearly fell over, laughing harder than any other moment in the two years we dated.

A few weeks later, she was listening as I wrapped up a phone call with a new business prospect, describing how we'd find each other in a coffeehouse. "I'm 6'1" and balding," I said. Edith giggled uncontrollably. "What?" I asked when I finished the call. "You told him you're balding," she said through her laugh. "Sweetie, you're not balding – you are *bald*." I knew it was funny, but I wasn't amused.

One of her favorite movies at that time was *Dangerous Liaisons* starring John Malkovich. She admitted that she had a bit of a crush on the actor and that when she first saw me, she thought I looked just like him. I was fine with that comparison, thinking I perhaps appealed to her bad-girl side. Nearly a dozen times when we dated, people would stare at me on the street, longer than I thought to be normal. I conjectured it was because I was bald and that made me look much older than I really was and they were wondering why an older man like me was dating an attractive younger woman such as Edith, though she was only four or five years my junior. She would notice the stares too and say, "They just think you're John Malkovich."

More often, I was a doppelgänger for the musician James Taylor. Though he is the age of my oldest brother, my receding hairline has tracked his, step for step. Once in the 1980s, I went to hear a concert at Charlotte's Double Door Inn by his younger brother, Livingston Taylor.

During a break, I noticed he wandered down a back hallway, opened a door and went in a room. I decided to follow him and, when I opened the door, I realized he had entered a back bar that was empty, save for the musician, sitting by himself at the bar, smoking a joint. I apologized, saying I didn't mean to interrupt his break and said I merely wanted to tell him how much I enjoyed his first set. He demurred, saying thanks and offered me a hit off his joint.

"I also wanted to tell you that people often stop me and say I look just like your brother James," I said.

"Dude, when you first walked in this bar, I did a double take, thinking he was busting me!" Livingston said.

I took that as strong confirmation of James' and my resemblance. A couple of years after Edith and I broke up, I went again to see the band GuruFish at Smith's Olde Bar in Midtown Atlanta. I did not see Edith there, though I perhaps was hoping for a similar outcome. A few minutes after I walked in and stood in the crowd, a man walked over.

"James Taylor!" he said. "Thanks so much for coming out to hear the band. It means so much to us. Would you mind joining the band onstage for a song?"

I took a moment to debate my circumstance. I may look like James Taylor, but I only spent a few weeks in high school trying to play a few James Taylor chords – and I absolutely cannot sing.

However, if I told him I wasn't James Taylor, he'd be embarrassed and even more important, disappointed. If I told him I was James Taylor, I'd be lying.

"Hey, I'm just here to listen to the band, but thanks," I said, figuring my presence would give the band something to talk about later in the green room.

"Well, at least let me buy you a beer!" the manager said. I spent less time pondering that response. "Sure," I said. I took the beer and hid myself in the back of the room.

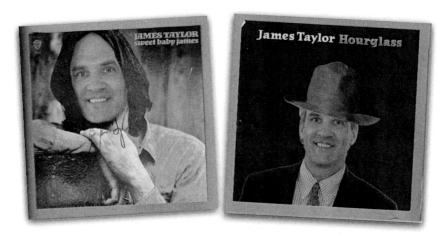

Age 49: My friends Jae Robbins and Jessica Childers at Resource Branding surprised me with a birthday card placing me in several James Taylor album covers.

Research says …

Three studies contribute to the literature on dominance and nonverbal behavior (Ellyson & Dovidio, 1985) by examining how a man's choice to shave his head influences person perception. In Study 1, men with shaved heads were rated as more dominant than similar men with full heads of hair. In Study 2, men whose hair was digitally removed were perceived as more dominant, taller, and stronger than their authentic selves. **Study 3 extends these results with nonphotographic stimuli and demonstrates how men experiencing natural hair loss may improve their interpersonal standing by shaving.** Theories of signaling, norm violation, and stereotypes are examined as explanations for the effect. Practical implications for men's psychological, social, and economic outlooks are also discussed.

– Mannes, Albert E.
"Shorn Scalps and Perceptions of Male Dominance."
Social Psychological and Personality Science 4, no. 2
(March 2013): 198–205. https://doi.org/
10.1177/1948550612449490.

7. Marrying Jan and Listening to Kevin

Since my sunburn episode, I've carefully put on sunscreen and worn a hat or cap whenever I go outside. Consequently, the top of my head has a healthy look, though the skin is very tender whenever I hit a low door frame, chandelier, or low-hanging tree branch. I grew more comfortable with my look as a bald man, though I haven't been pleased to see the open area continue to enlarge through the years. Twice, as the hair retreated lower, it has revealed red spots that hid below the hair. Dermatologists have diagnosed them as seborrheic keratoses, benign growths that they easily removed by freezing with liquid nitrogen or minor surgery. Fortunately, the skin heals rather quickly, though such procedures performed on areas under existing hair follicles often result in those hairs departing permanently.

I was married the first time for 13 years, was single for 13 years, and have been married for the second time to a lovely woman named Jan since 2005. She's a travel writer and I get to accompany her occasionally on her trips. Whenever we take selfies, she always comments on whether it shows her "good side" or if her hair is in place. I don't think she has a bad side and she has wonderful blonde hair that always provides a stark contrast to my bald head. I don't often have a comment on how she looks because I was

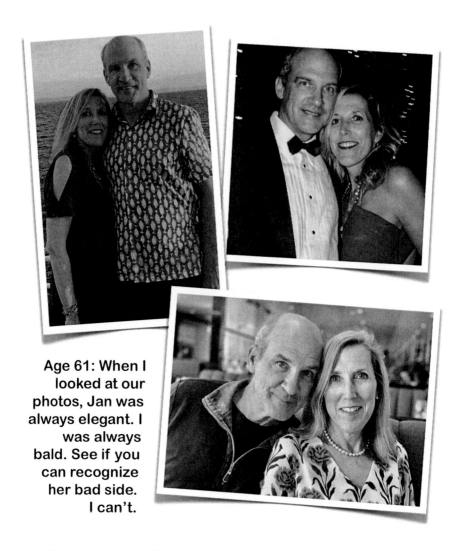

Age 61: When I looked at our photos, Jan was always elegant. I was always bald. See if you can recognize her bad side. I can't.

usually gazing at my lightbulb of a head, wishing I had half the hair she does. I also had the pleasure of getting to know Jan's dad and he had a respectable head of hair. That reassured me that she loves me for who I am and not because I resembled her dad.

Before we got married, Jan and her daughter Catherine went shopping for her wedding dress. As they were checking out, a young sales clerk behind the counter was talking about a book she was reading that mentioned aliens.

"The premise of the book is there are aliens already living amongst us," the woman said. "They look like regular humans, but they are always bald and wear glasses."

Jan burst out laughing and told the group at the cash register, "Oh my gosh. I'm marrying an alien!"

Jan doesn't understand the James Taylor lookalike and often shakes her head when friends or passersby bring it up. Once, on a travel writers' trip to the Quebec Winter Carnival, we were having dinner with other travel writers when a woman from the next table kept staring at me. I was flattered, though Jan may have been annoyed. Before we settled the bill, the woman walked over to speak to me.

"Has anyone ever told you …" she began.

"Yes, I know, you think I look like James Taylor," I said.

"No," she said. "You don't understand. I'm James Taylor's yoga teacher. You are a spitting image of him."

Jan looked at me and said, "Well that's pretty strong confirmation."

It was during my marriage to Jan that I began walking down to the neighborhood barber, West Barber Shop, a much fancier barber shop than old Mr. Evans'. Its proprietor, Kevin Serani, had bought the business recently and was happy to welcome me as a new client. He understood when I told him I liked what little hair remained to look as full and long as possible, though I'd agree to let him trim it above my ears and collar. When I first started going to Kevin, his going rate was $15. I observed when I waited in a

chair for him, he'd labor much longer over other customers'
haircuts while mine would take less than 10 minutes.

"I think you should charge me less than your other clients," I'd
joke with Kevin. "I have less hair and you're finished with me in
five minutes."

"No, no," Kevin would say. "You don't understand. Yours is
more difficult. The hairs on the back and sides of your head are
very, very thick and then I must find those occasional hairs on top
of your head and clip them."

Kevin also began trying to talk me into becoming one of his
special clients – those who, like me, had no hair on top but lots on
the sides.

"I take clients several times a year to Istanbul, Turkey, and
accompany them to a famous doctor there. He can move your hair
follicles from the side and put them on top and you'll have a full
head of hair again!"

"Kevin," I'd always respond, "I'm too old for that. Besides, it
would all just fall out again. And my mother would be furious. She
threatens to snatch any fake hair off the top of my head."

"But it wouldn't be fake," he'd say. "It would be your natural
hair, just moved up top."

This same conversation went on for years. In 2016, my mother,
Van Spalding Schroder, died at age 99 and I began pondering the
validity of Kevin's suggested change to my look.

"Why Istanbul?" I asked one day.

"Turkey is the center of the world for hair transplantation,"
Kevin said. "The doctors there are much further ahead of the
doctors anywhere else. They've perfected the technique. People fly
there from all over the world to have their hair transplanted. I'm
telling you, Chris, you would look amazing. You will look so much
younger and you'll be so much happier. Come with me this fall on

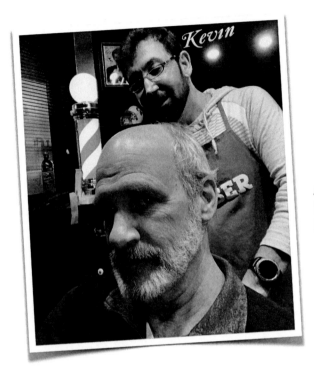

Age 62: Kevin
Serani had
been pitching
me for years to
go with him to
Istanbul.
In 2019, it
just started
sounding like a
better idea.

my trip. It's five days, you only pay $5,000, he'll move 5,000 hair follicles and that includes airfare, your stay in a five-star hotel, dinner in five-star restaurants, and I'll personally give you a tour of all the amazing historical sites in Istanbul."

After leaving the newspaper business, I had started my own PR firm, primarily serving commercial real estate (CRE) developers, architects, financial, and legal clients, leading that successfully for nearly two decades. Business development meant attending one or two networking events a week, convincing mostly older white guys to allow my firm to raise their profile in the media.

Over time, I added a team, landing eventually on a formula of hiring bright young female graduates of college PR programs. It wasn't that I chose to hire women – it just turned out that PR programs graduated many women and relatively few men. I eventually promoted one woman, Sarah Funderburk Weston, to partner and she and I would attend networking events together. I noticed over time that the younger generation of CRE pros gravitated to talking with her. And the older guys weren't unhappy about that choice either.

In 2012, a PR firm owner named Charlie Hayslett who was 10 years older than me asked me to lunch. "Chris, when you get into your mid-sixties like I am, people start to look at you differently. They see me and they say, 'he's just an old guy about to retire.'

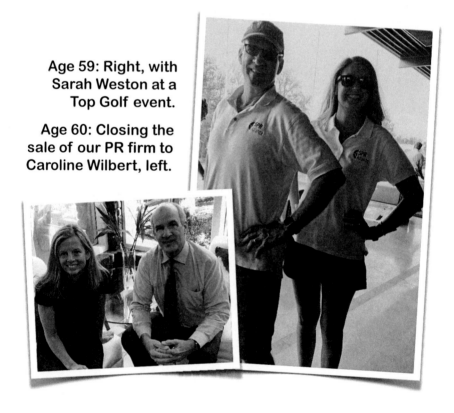

Age 59: Right, with Sarah Weston at a Top Golf event.

Age 60: Closing the sale of our PR firm to Caroline Wilbert, left.

They don't want to hire me anymore." Charlie's words
reverberated with me. When I looked at him, he had a full head of
gray hair and short gray beard. It only reinforced my fears of how
people were assessing my looks.

In 2017, a woman named Caroline Wilbert who had started a PR
firm in Atlanta with her husband and who'd tried to recruit Sarah
to their firm, stopped me at a CRE networking gala and asked me
to lunch. She and her husband had divorced the year before. She
had bought him out and her client portfolio was growing quickly.
At lunch the next week, she said she'd like to buy my PR firm,
taking my employees and my clients.

"Would you want me to join your firm?" I asked.

"Goodness, no," she said. "I just finished buying out my
husband. I don't need another old guy around telling me what to
do."

I laughed. For a moment, I considered if I should be offended.
Then I realized her timing was perfect. Two years earlier, I had
started a second business based on a newsletter and website
business that my PR firm helped launch for a group of journalists
who'd taken buyouts from the daily paper. Tweaking that concept
to feature shorter stories of exactly 100-word lengths, I was
spending half my time flying to other cities, recruiting new clients
for my firm, The 100 Companies, while also running the PR firm
with Sarah's help. I concluded I was probably doing a poor job of
running both firms. Two months later, I sold Caroline my PR firm.

In the spring of 2019, I visited Kevin again for a haircut. As
always, he finished the appointment trying to sell me on going to
Istanbul. By then, his price has increased to $7,000, but since I had
some cash from my PR firm sale, I lingered and asked more
details. As I walked home, I reflected on what Charlie and Caroline
had said in prior years. I also thought about my newsletter business

and the fact most of my sales prospects were agency owners – primarily women in their thirties or forties – who led even younger teammates. When I walked into their conference rooms for the first time, I often feared their first thoughts they said to themselves were, "He's old – and bald." I reasoned that if I agreed to go with Kevin to Istanbul, then these prospects would then only say, "He's old," and that might improve my sales results. One of the secrets to sales, after all, is to remove as many obstacles to closing as possible.

When I got home I told Jan, as I had several times before, that Kevin said I should go with him to Istanbul. This time, instead of saying nothing or saying, "That's crazy," she thought for a moment and said rather softly, "That might be interesting. I've never seen you with hair."

"Really," I said?

"Really," she said.

And so began my serious consideration of moving my hair.

Research says ...

In order to investigate the relationship between male hair loss and psychological distress, 182 men were recruited who had a wide range of ages and hair loss varying from none to severe. Care was taken to ensure that hair loss and age were uncorrelated in the sample. Multiple regression was used to predict possible consequences of baldness, controlling for age, and examining the interaction between baldness and age to see if consequences were especially severe in cases of premature baldness.

Increasing degrees of hair loss were associated with loss of self-esteem, depression, introversion, neuroticism and feeling unattractive. These effects were more marked for young men in the case of self-esteem, introversion and feeling unattractive.

*– Wells PA, Willmoth T, Russell RJ.
Does fortune favour the bald?
Psychological correlates of hair loss in males.
Br J Psychol. August 1995*

8. Going to Istanbul

A few days later, as I drove Jan to the airport for one of her trips, she pulled out her iPhone and asked the name of the Turkish doctor. Scrolling photos, she became more intrigued. "I think you should consider doing it," she said. "It might be fun but I think you should first talk to people Kevin's taken there already." After dropping her off at the airport, I called Kevin and told him to hold me a spot on his late October trip and I asked for names of previous clients.

"I wish I had done it a long time ago," the first client said. "I'm only in my thirties and I'm not totally bald, but my hairline has been receding and thinning for a while. About six months after I returned, I went to a wedding and all my friends kept looking at my head, but they didn't say anything. Looking at your photo, I think the difference will be much more dramatic and your friends will react instantly."

That's what I was counting on. When I told Steve Massell, a friend I'd known since high school, what I was considering, he looked at me for a few moments and issued his verdict: "No, that's not the Chris we know and love. Don't do it." When I revealed my plans to my two children, Sally and Thomas, over dinner, they fell silent. They didn't remember me with hair and the concept was almost too foreign for them to respond. When I told restaurateur friend Tom Murphy, he reacted positively, so much so, he committed to going with me just so he could experience Istanbul.

"I've always wanted to go," he said.

When Tom and his wife Susan came over for dinner a few weeks later, I kidded Susan, putting my arm around Tom's shoulder, looking at his robust head of white hair, saying, "Susan, it was so nice of Tom to volunteer to be my hair donor." She and Tom looked at each other in shock and started laughing. Later that evening, he bailed on joining me. "I'm afraid I'm going to wake up in Istanbul bald and without a kidney!" he said.

When I told my brother, Mike, he also said he wanted to join me – not to have his hair transplanted, though his hair has thinned in the past few years, but because of Kevin's offer to provide a tour of Istanbul's historic sites.

The last time Mike was in Turkey, his trip was interrupted. It was July 1974 and he was the sole travel guide for 28 college women on a summer European tour. Half the group of women touring the Hagia Sophia were bored and wanted to sneak away to go shopping at the Grand Bazaar. The local tour guide was offended, cut off the tour, led the group back to the bus, and began berating them over the speaker. The guide was then notified that Greece had just declared war on Turkey and had invaded the disputed island of Cyprus.

Mike's primary concern became getting his increasingly hysterical students back to their Greek ship, moored in the Turkish harbor, before it departed early without them. When they arrived at port, the Greek crew was frantically waving passengers on board and just as Mike's group walked up the ramp, the crew gave a suitcase full of passports to the harbormaster, and told them to send the other American passengers they were leaving behind to the

Age 62: With my skeptical friends …

Top: Tom and Susan Murphy.

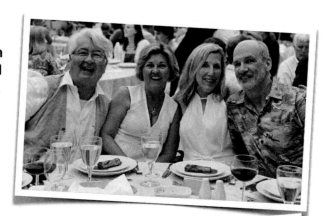

Center: Ken Smith, Norris Broyles, and David Martin.

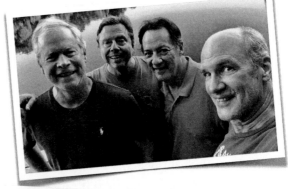

Below: me, Norris Broyles, Tom Murphy, Ken Smith, Steve Massell, Mike Egan, Charles Driebe, and Dennis Zakas.

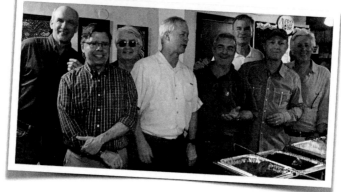

U.S. embassy. The Greek ship turned its lights off and quietly glided out of the harbor as war planes buzzed overhead.

"I've always wanted to finish my tour of the Hagia Sophia," Mike said.

Since Kevin first mentioned Istanbul, I was curious as to why Turkey, of all places, had become the world's center for hair transplant surgery. Since my return from there, on the rare occasion I've told my story, people were more intrigued with the Istanbul angle than why I had follicle surgery in the first place.

As to the latter, they are missing the point. For decades, I missed having my hair. Though no one other than my mother ever asked me about it, I sensed a chronic difference separating me from other men as if I were missing an ear or a finger. I thought being bald was the first element people noticed about me and it was the primary one they filed away in their memory to help recognize me.

In all other ways, I felt complete as a man, except for the prominent absence of hair atop my head. I was proud of how I bounced back from a gauntlet of personal losses in my mid-thirties – divorced from what I'd hoped to be a lifelong marriage, fired from what I thought was my dream job, shaken by the death of my father, and separated from my children when my ex-wife re-married and moved to her new husband's hometown of Charlotte.

I eventually re-kindled the confidence and momentum that I'd lost in the latter years of my marriage to my first wife. I left my job, started my own neighborhood newspaper, and dated lovely, self-confident women, eventually meeting the love of my life, Jan. As I succeeded somewhat as an entrepreneur, I deepened the relationship with my two children, continued the cultivation of friends, spirituality, and my faith in God. I became more accepting of my appearance and my goal of making my way in the world, focusing on being kind.

As to the former, why go to Istanbul: I had considered solutions to my hair loss, but I was ever-skeptical. I was keenly aware of imperfect attempts to repair male pattern baldness, spotting guys who perhaps had a bad experience with replacement. One neighbor had dark hair plugs, a solution that was preferred through the 1970s. He always wears a cap.

Recently, a relative tried a newer technique called strip harvesting – developed in the 1980s that moved a full section of hair from the back of the head to the front – with unhappy results. I had seen print ads, television commercials, and billboards for hair transplant facilities in the USA, but I had grown to accept the bald life was my destiny. Yet Kevin always assured me the relatively newer method of follicular unit extraction (FUE), in which individual follicles are removed with a special punch scalpel, was the way to go.

He assured me that visiting Istanbul and this doctor was best for me for several reasons – it was more affordable, the medical procedures are more advanced there, and the city was a beautiful place to visit. He would tell me during my years of barbershop visits that Istanbul doctors had evaluated research and developed methods that were more advanced than other countries, including the USA. It didn't seem logical to me, so I did a little research.

As with all medical advances, online literature catalogs an evolving debate as to the causes of male pattern baldness – and to solutions to reversing it. A preferred theory for decades was that men were likely to grow bald if their maternal grandfather was follicly challenged. My maternal grandfather had an enviable head of dark hair and yet my paternal grandfather was bald – so I didn't believe that old wives' tale. Later, research suggested that a combination of certain regional gene pools (Northern European, Caribbean, and Middle Eastern) with a high level of testosterone led to hair loss. That worked for me, I could tell people I had lots of testosterone.

Deeper research proffered the cause was a combination of testosterone binding with and converting into a more potent yet natural hormone called dihydrotestosterone (DHT). DHT causes skin and fat surrounding hair follicles to shrink, squeezing the environment surrounding a shaft of hair until the follicle shrinks and eventually falls out, never to return.

Perhaps a more important discovery was that it wasn't the environment where the hair grew and from which it disappeared, but rather the genetic makeup of the cells of the hairs that grew there. In other words, most balding men still have hair around the middle of their heads and research showed that side-of-the-head hair had a different genetic makeup than hair on top of the head. If carefully and meticulously transplanted employing FUE, the theory went, this side hair didn't react so adversely to the chemical stew of testosterone and DHT and would instead grow healthily for years where other "native" hair had failed.

Technology improved alongside the research, with the introduction of smaller punch blades that surround and lift the follicle out of its original location as well as microscopic blades that cut into the skin to make a place for its new home.

As far as I can understand and surmise, Istanbul became a world leader in hair transplantation due to a curious confluence of economic forces. The first is simple – cost. While the FUE procedure in the USA can cost between $10,000 and $20,000 in Atlanta, the same – Kevin would argue much better – procedure would cost you $2,000 to $5,000 in Istanbul.

This is partly attributed to Turkey's cost of living, which is much lower than in the USA or U.K. Second, its supply of expertise is greater. In the 1980s, a group of Istanbul doctors seized the

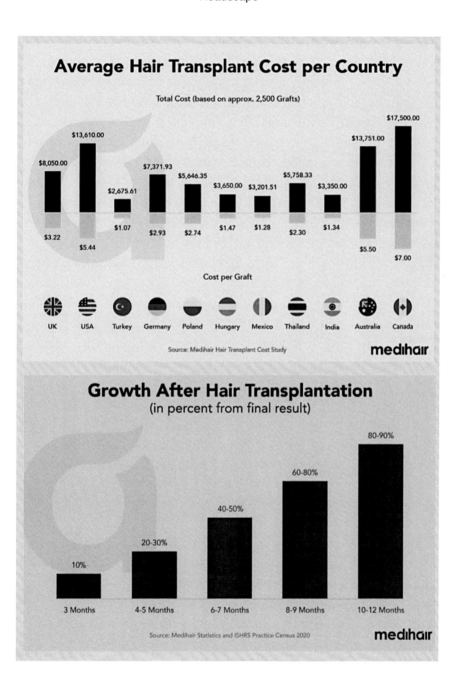

Average Hair Transplant Cost per Country

Total Cost (based on approx. 2,500 Grafts)

- UK: $8,050.00 — $3.22
- USA: $13,610.00 — $5.44
- Turkey: $2,675.61 — $1.07
- Germany: $7,371.93 — $2.93
- Poland: $5,646.35 — $2.74
- Hungary: $3,650.00 — $1.47
- Mexico: $3,201.51 — $1.28
- Thailand: $5,758.33 — $2.30
- India: $3,350.00 — $1.34
- Australia: $13,751.00 — $5.50
- Canada: $17,500.00 — $7.00

Cost per Graft

UK USA Turkey Germany Poland Hungary Mexico Thailand India Australia Canada

Source: Medihair Hair Transplant Cost Study

medihair

Growth After Hair Transplantation
(in percent from final result)

- 3 Months: 10%
- 4-5 Months: 20-30%
- 6-7 Months: 40-50%
- 8-9 Months: 60-80%
- 10-12 Months: 80-90%

Source: Medihair Statistics and ISHRS Practice Census 2020

medihair

opportunity to specialize in this practice area and began competing against each other. Their success generated a wave of interest in the procedure – not only among prospective patients but also from other physicians, medical students, and a growing class of well-trained and highly skilled medical technicians who exponentially enlarged the supply of expertise – and drove down its cost.

This growing tourism revenue caught the attention of less-reputable practitioners, who offered lower prices for less-successful and less-safe procedures. It also attracted the Turkish government, which began to regulate the reported $1 billion industry to protect its tax revenue and the industry's reputation. They began closing hair clinics that did not meet standards set by the Turkish Ministry of Health.

Combine Turkey's total medical tourism industry, which has grown from $1.5 billion in 2018 to an expected $20 billion in 2023, with it being headquarters to Turkish Airlines, which serves the most countries (121) of any airline and 30 more than its closest competitor (Air France).

Finally, Turkey opened its new international airport on October 29, 2018 on the European side of Istanbul. The first phase included the largest footprint of any airport terminal under one roof (15 million square feet) and, after it completes four more phases at a total overall cost of $12 billion by 2025, it will have eight runways, 16 taxiways and an expected annual passenger count of 150 million.

Almost one year after its opening, on Saturday, October 26, 2019, Kevin, Mike, and I were flying into IST on the nearly 11-hour nonstop flight from Atlanta. I was scheduled for surgery in Istanbul on Monday morning. Kevin was a dozen rows away. Trying to induce sleep for the overnight journey, Mike and I ordered and enjoyed several drinks from the complimentary alcoholic beverage cart. A few hours later, Kevin wandered back and saw how much fun we were having.

"Chris, you aren't drinking are you?" Kevin asked.

"Of course," I said.

"I don't think you can drink alcohol for 48 hours before surgery," Kevin said. I was not happy.

"You never told me," I protested. When we landed, Kevin called the clinic, confirming the restriction (alcohol and tobacco reduce chances of success) and moving not only my surgery one day later to Tuesday, but our flight back home two days later. The extra days allowed me to keep the mandatory 48-hour follow-up appointment to ensure there was no infection and to remove my bandages – and to book the only available non-stop flight back home.

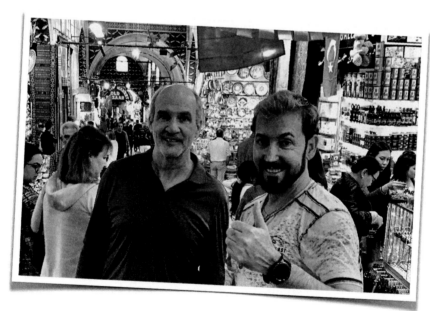

At Istanbul's Grand Bazaar with Kevin.

"Don't worry, Chris," Kevin said. "This way, you and Mike will get to see more of Istanbul." That we did.

Nevertheless, after landing in Istanbul and checking in the hotel, I had a sudden unexpected drop in energy and enthusiasm. Perhaps it was what seemed to be a developing head cold, or perhaps it was the jet lag or the fact I can't sleep on a plane or the sudden realization that my brother Mike and I weren't going to have the few days of adventure together that I had envisioned – the only trip I've ever taken with just one of my four siblings – a venture that was to include wine and beers.

In addition, Kevin had implied that following surgery I may have to take Propecia and that also might conflict with alcohol. I began to research it during our flight and the results were not promising. While it was primarily helpful to stop or reverse hair loss, it also helped with enlarged prostate glands. It was the side effects that bothered me most. Those included an inability to have or maintain an erection, decreased sexual desire, problems with ejaculation, pain in the testicles, and depression. Reading those was enough to kick in those side effects in me before I even started taking it.

As we passed the Duty Free shop in the impressive, brand new, expansive Istanbul airport, Mike grabbed a bottle of bourbon, then apologized because I couldn't share it.

"Oh, you should buy it and drink it," I said. "I just wish Kevin had told me ahead of this trip that I wouldn't be able to drink. I hadn't planned for that."

And yet, that mood slid that evening into a deepening sense of buyer's remorse. I wondered if this whole trip was folly and that I was wasting my time and money. Before going to bed, I wrote my wife Jan a frustrated email:

"Radisson Blu is nice but room is hot and we can't seem to fix that. Not sleeping well. I hear now I may have hair for a few weeks and then it falls out for a few months. I don't know. Plus I have to take Propecia for three months and that reduces sex-ability and drive. Fighting stupid cold. Mike is having fun even if I'm not so much. Wondering if I made right decision doing this. Kevin keeps telling me I'm going to look totally different. But I'm feeling tired and old and a bit depressed and am wondering why I'm doing this at 62? Been awake for a couple hours and can't have a drink and second guessing myself on everything."

Jan, the ever-supportive wife, sent a cheery email from a Cabo San Lucas resort where she was on a travel writers' trip.

"Oh I'm sorry. Can you switch rooms? I would ask. Sorry to hear about side effects, but it's only three months. But Kevin should have given you more information. Maybe tell Kevin about your doubts about all of it? But you are not too old to do this – you have decades left to enjoy your hair. But too bad about the not drinking thing, which he also should have told you about. I'm sorry – things will look better when you get sleep."

Despite my cold and sour mood, Istanbul itself was fascinating – a blend of ancient walls, some erected by the Roman Emperor Constantine in the fourth century – shadowing a modern city that straddled a breathtaking body of water named the Bosporus that divided the city's footprint on both the European and Asian continents. Kevin was in love with Istanbul and though Mike and I had each briefly visited before, Kevin's enthusiasm sparked a growing fascination in Mike and me. The city's population had nearly doubled in the previous 20 years.

Kevin paid to maneuver us to the front of many of the lines outside several historic mosques, museums, and finally, the Hagia Sophia. He also took us to the Grand Bazaar, which combines two things I hate more than anything – shopping and bargaining – with another: hawkers who try to entice you into their lairs. Kevin bought some custom-blended vitamin-infused honey from one vendor and then we escaped for a wonderful boat tour of the city from the Bosporus. Later that afternoon, Kevin introduced us to friends he had developed in previous trips – native Turks with whom he was negotiating to launch hair studios that could steer more clients to him and the Estefirst Clinic.

When Kevin checked us into the hotel, he made sure we found our way to the hotel restaurant, which was better than we expected. The only part of Kevin's promised tour on which he didn't deliver was taking us to the city's restaurants – he was distracted by his friends and business partners – but Mike and I found our way fine through the historic streets of Istanbul.

One night, as we stood on a busy street trying to understand why we couldn't find a restaurant we selected on Tripadvisor, a nicely dressed gentleman tried to get our attention, saying, "Guys, guys!" We ignored him until he persisted and walked right up to us, asking how he could help. It turned out Recep Cok really was trying to provide assistance. He was a fascinating person. He walked us to a kebab restaurant he recommended over those in Tripadvisor, which he claimed was not reliable in many countries, including Turkey. "It's all sponsored here," he said. "It's crap. You have to rely on locals like me for authentic recommendations."

At dinner, Recep, who had great hair, introduced us to other locals and suggested excellent selections from the menu. He then invited us to his and his wife Michelle's home, where he proudly showed us his stunning collection of Turkish rugs, tapestries, and art that he curated in his four-story home. We were so happy to have met him.

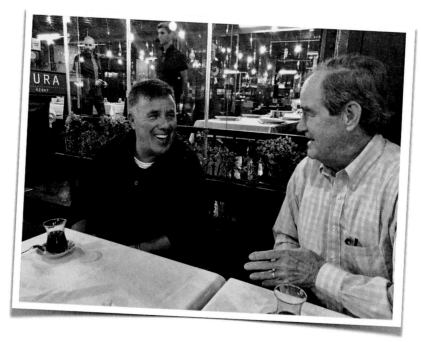

Recep Cok, left, stopped me and Mike, right, on the historic streets of Istanbul, escorted us to his recommended restaurant and gave us a sneak peak of his art collection.

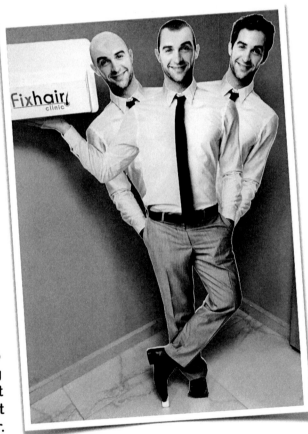

The standup poster walking into meet Göksal said it all: Fixhair.

9. Göksal and the "Fixhair" Clinic

O n the day of my surgical appointment, Kevin drove us a few miles away to a healthcare district where Göksal Öztürk's office was set up. I was a little nervous at first. We tried to park in a small lot squeezed in front of two buildings on a busy street, but it was full, so Kevin negotiated with an attendant while Mike and I waited inside the building lobby. It didn't appear to be a hospital exactly, but there were a number of healthcare-related businesses operating on the first floor. Finally, Kevin returned, led us down a hallway and down a flight of stairs to a basement space.

At first I didn't recognize it as the Estefirst office as there was no branded entrance door and a number of doors were closed to what I learned were appointment rooms. The hallway was painted a medium to dark gray color. I noted a stand-up cardboard cutout against one wall that showed a man with three heads: one bald, one with some hair, and one with a thick covering. It featured two English words: "Fixhair clinic."

I was intrigued how these physicians in Istanbul, with English as their second language, could concisely describe what to me had been such a complicated decision – interwoven with a half lifetime of emotion, drama, and insecurity – into one simple word: fixhair.

It reduced all my angst to one simple proposition: my hair might have been broken for three decades, but in a matter of hours, they were going to do what one does when anything breaks – you just fix it.

This was not a slick, suburban, upscale healthcare spa in America where one might pay two to ten times more and hope for the best. This was an efficient, Eurasian clinic where dozens of successful medical procedures were completed each week by professional medical personnel who did nothing else day in and day out. As I ventured deeper into the clinic, I concluded the practice had expanded from a series of rooms at the end of the basement hallway, growing back towards the stairway door through which we had entered. I was visiting in October 2019. Göksal's and Dr. Aslan's medical practice has since moved to a larger, nicer space in the Şişli section of Istanbul. In their busy seasons, when they book more clients than they have procedure rooms to serve, they will occasionally lease extra rooms from nearby hospitals.

Kevin recognized one of the technicians and told her we were there for our appointment. She said Göksal was on a phone call, but would be with us shortly. When he walked out and introduced himself, I was surprised – he was younger than I expected, but I could see from the photos on his desk that he was married and had a young son. He had a head of dark hair and a short beard. He exuded a friendly, yet solid confidence combined with a joyful personality that instantly put me at ease. His facility with English was less than fluent but more than adequate to discuss what I should expect that day and beyond.

Turns out, Göksal is an anesthetist and the chief of the team and not, as Kevin may have implied, a doctor. Kevin is an endearing salesperson, so I can't blame him for some inflation.

Göksal introduced us to his staff, several young, friendly, and professionally dressed associates. His physician, Dr. Veli Aslan, was not there that week. Dr. Aslan was one of the first to practice hair transplantation in Turkey, back when they deployed the old FUT method.

Mike and Kevin accompanied me to a back room where Göksal explained the sequence of that day's procedure. They took my blood pressure, looked me over, drew some blood, and sent part of the sample to be tested to ensure I was HIV-negative.

Göksal grabbed a marker and outlined the contours on my forehead where my hairs would be moved. His markings defined the border between the skin pores that would continue to be bare

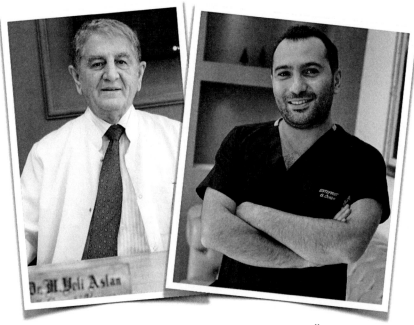

Dr. Veli Aslan and Anesthetist Göksal Öztürk

and the ones that would be devoted to nurturing my new crop of mostly gray hair. His design, with a region veering out over the middle of my forehead, seemed too good to be true. The last time I had hair there, it was a peninsula, or Two Mile Island. Now it would be part of a substantive land grab that would change the course of my appearance and, perhaps my personal history.

His team then shaved my hair to a tiny fraction of an inch – a length that would make it easier to extract and replant the follicles. I asked him to wait while I got out of the chair and looked at myself in a mirror. I was shocked. I had never seen myself with extremely short hair. Though all the follicles had fallen off the top of my head, I had always been blessed with thick hair around the sides and I had been mindful to keep what hair I had as thick as possible.

I had noticed in the previous decade the trend among men who had begun to lose their hair to instead completely shave their heads, showing no hair. I didn't ever understand that style, though I did think it was most attractive on Black men like Michael Jordan and other NBA players and analysts. I had never considered shaving my head. Now, having my head nearly shaved bald for the first time, I was stunned that it actually looked sharp. For the second time since arriving in Istanbul, I began to question the wisdom of proceeding with the follicle surgery.

"I look cool," I said, rubbing my layer of short, stubbly hair. Mike and Kevin agreed. "Maybe I should just wear it like this and then I won't need to transplant them to the top."

"No way," Kevin said, gently pushing me back in the chair, laughing. "You're going to be so happy when you do this, Chris. Trust me." After the four of us agreed on the schedule, we took some photos and then Kevin and Mike left. I spent the next six hours with Göksal and his medical staff.

The next step in the process was to inject what they call the "donor area" of my scalp with a local anesthetic to remove any possibility of pain during and after surgery. Göksal asked about my alcohol and tobacco intake as that can affect the amount of anesthesia they inject. I wasn't a smoker and it had been two days since I had alcohol, so I was ready for the recommended dosage. Then, following a generous round of tiny injections around the sides of my head that rendered the donor region numb, the real work began.

In normal situations, Dr. Aslan or Göksal might perform the initial stages of surgery and then move from room to room to supervise other procedures going on simultaneously, but Kevin had impressed upon Göksal that I was a special patient with a large

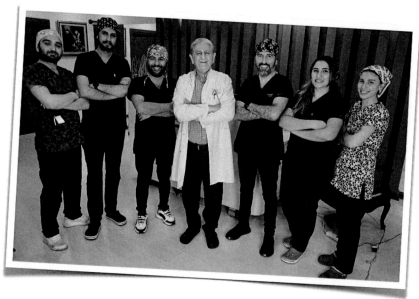

The clinic team in their new 2022 offices.

group of bald friends who could later become patients. Kevin urged him to perform the surgery himself, which he happily did. Kevin had earlier been a patient of Estefirst and was pleased with how his follicles were transplanted to offset his own receding hairline.

For nearly three hours that morning, as I leaned back in a surgical chair that left my scalp exposed for their work, Göksal and a male colleague employed a device called a microfue that is equipped with synthetic saffire that is harder and more precise than a steel blade. It enables them to encircle each graft, making a small incision into my scalp to encapsulate the roots, and remove my follicles. With each incision, they are able to capture one to three follicles in each graft, comprising what they call a nest.

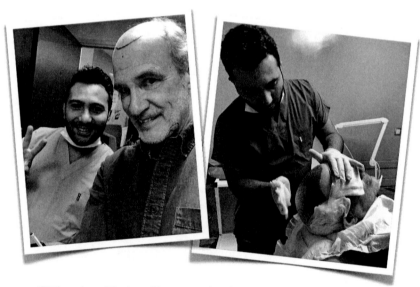

Göksal outlining the surgical areas and patting me down after a day of surgery in his Istanbul clinic.

Although my band of hair around the sides and back of my head was thick as Kevin discovered, the medical staff asked after they reached a count of 4,000 if they could instead begin harvesting some of the hairs from my beard below my jaw to fill in the area at the crown of my scalp where most men have a bald spot. Since I am 6'1", they suggested most people seeing me from the front would never see that area anyway. As that might enable me to shave less often under my jawline, I invited them to take as many as they'd like. They stopped at an overall count of 5,000, leaving many hairs on my neck to shave in the future. They kept those separated from the other hairs that had been growing on the sides of my head. (This turned out to be a smart move as later, the beard hairs seem to grow in with less discipline than the others.)

When they finished harvesting, they invited me to view what Göksal affectionately called "your babies" soaking in an isotonic solution, lined up in straight rows in several metal trays. To this solution they added some platelet-rich plasma (php) that was processed from a unit of my blood that they extracted before surgery. The php is believed to help increase the thickness of the hair shaft. I looked at my babies, resting on pieces of cloth. They looked hauntingly like small filets of salmon. I was worried about how long they would be on their own in the trays, but Göksal assured me they would be fine while his staff served me a nice lunch of rice, meat, and vegetables in the reception area.

After lunch, it was planting time. They led me back into the same appointment room and injected more anesthesia, but this time they applied it to the transplant area. They applied pressure on the top of my head and found a few spots were still sensitive, so they injected more anesthetic. When they were confident the anesthetic was working well, they began reversing the earlier procedure – instead of extracting hair follicles, they spent the next three hours planting them in rows around the area outlined on my scalp. During the afternoon, this procedure was performed by Göksal and one or two of his female technicians. This time, their method of punching in small holes in my head to plant my follicles did register more of a sound, something I likened to listening inside a melon while small punctures were made to its rind.

It was a strange, but not unpleasant sound that I heard for nearly three hours, overlaid with a continuous conversation between the doctor and his technicians. They spoke in Turkish and I was left to imagine what they talked about as they changed the course of my history. Were they talking about the latest Netflix downloads or was it medically oriented – or were they gossiping about their families? I was left to dream about what I might look like in a few months until their constant punch-and-plant sounds were complete. Göksal said they planted my hair at a 40- or 45-degree angle, so when I parted my hair across my head the way I used to three decades ago, it would fall in the natural direction. However, he said I could comb it in any direction I wanted. Comb – that was an item I had not used in 30 years.

The most amazing part of the surgery was how I never felt any pain in such a sensitive area of my head. No doubt, the anesthetic did its job, but the latest precision equipment as well as the skill and confidence of Göksal and his team were equally responsible. He estimated his clinic had performed 20,000 similar surgeries since 2008.

"When we started performing hair transplant surgery, there were only a few clinics here and perhaps 40 to 50 experts who participated in the surgeries," Göksal said. "Experience is important. You learn something in each operation." There are many, many more practitioners in Turkey now.

I heard Kevin's voice outside the room near the end of my procedure. He knocked on the door to ask how I was doing and I assured him I was fine. Göksal carefully blotted what little beads of blood appeared on my scalp with a cloth before wrapping that day's work with some soft cotton gauze and finished my "turban" with a few bands of tape. He then gave me a few sample boxes of "vitamins" as he called them and instructed me to replenish them with a larger supply there in Istanbul or back in the USA.

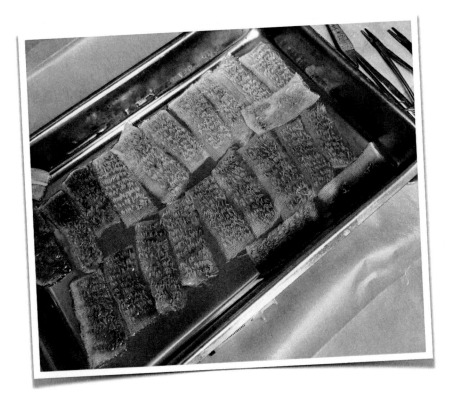

My "babies" soaking while I enjoyed a nice Turkish lunch.

Before leaving for Istanbul, I had talked with a few men who had invested in hair transplants in the USA at some brand-name clinics that advertised on television and they all described being prescribed a handful of post-surgical drugs. I asked Göksal about taking those painkillers or perhaps even some hair growth hormones such as Propecia or Rogaine which I had always heard about but never taken.

"Please, no," Göksal said. "Do not take those drugs. All you need now are these vitamins, but please take them every day for 90 days. No other medicine needed." I looked at the samples and researched their ingredients and how to order them back home. I was intrigued to find out the pills, Priorin, were comprised of biotin, or vitamin B7, as well as millet, which I remembered as an old-world grain mentioned in the Bible and ancient literature. I also remembered it was a primary ingredient of my favorite snack bar that was comprised of several seed grains. I had eaten one or two of these seed bars daily for several years and asked if it was acceptable to continue eating them along with his pills.

"Priorin is really all you need," Göksal said. "We found it contains nutrients that are perfect for newly planted hair follicles. It goes directly to strengthen your hair follicles but after this initial dosage, we don't believe they provide any continuing benefit to hair in general. The procedure that each doctor considers appropriate after surgery may be different. We decide with our experience from more than 20 years … who used what, how much, what effect … these examples guide our people."

I asked about wearing a cap or hat to hide the bandages on my head and Göksal shook his head. "Hats are no good for hair," he said. "Hair needs lots of air and just a little sunlight to grow back in. The humidity under a hat is not good for its progress."

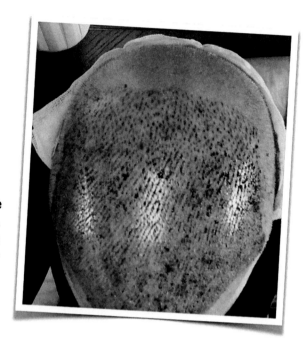

My scalp at the end of the day. 5,000 follicles spending their first night in their new homeland.

He instructed Kevin that we should return in 48 hours for a mandatory progress check and to remove my bandages. Meanwhile, Kevin continued giving me and Mike a tour of Istanbul's sights. I was at first insecure about wearing my head bandages, thinking people might think I had an accident or brain surgery. However, just as Kevin predicted, we saw many more men walking the streets of Istanbul with the same bandages on.

The next day, I visited a pharmacy in downtown Istanbul and bought a 90-day supply of Priorin. I checked out and turned to step down the short staircase back to street level. A lovely brunette was walking up the stairs and, when she looked at me and my bandages, she gave me a very welcoming smile as if she recognized me. "Could my new look be having my desired affect already, even with bandages still on?" I asked myself. I smiled back broadly and said hello. Then I noticed her husband walking a couple of steps behind. He had the same crown of bandages around his head. The three of us enjoyed a tribal-bonding laugh.

On the second afternoon, Kevin drove me back to Göksal's office and they removed my bandages, poured some warm water and an anti-bacterial solution over the red spots on my scalp, gently blotted them with a towel and, after an inspection of my tiny wounds, announced that we were good to go. He supplied me with a few days of antibiotics, pain relievers and a shampoo that had a surgery-specific pH value of 5.5.

"I'm sure Kevin told you," Göksal explained, "that your hair follicles are taking root in your skin, but that they've been through a great deal of trauma. They will be fine, but don't be alarmed in the coming weeks when your hair falls out and you are again bald. The roots are still there and the follicles will grow back a few weeks later. In a year, you will have a full head of hair, as long as you take these vitamins for 90 days and nothing else. And try not to wear hats or pull your clothes over your head for the first few weeks."

"I'm not going to let my hair fall out, Göksal," I said. "I plan on keeping them." He laughed, saying that in rare cases, much of the hair does remain, but not to be alarmed when it falls out at first, as almost always happens with transplant cases. "It's natural," he said.

Amazingly, I never needed to take the pain relievers as I never felt any pain. I did fret about my scalp for days, though. I worried about lying on a pillow, fearing it would rub the follicles out. I worried about putting on a hat when I briefly needed to shield the sun, thinking it would not allow the hair to breathe. When I inevitably bumped my head on a wall in the hotel room, I ran to the mirror to make sure all the follicles were still there.

They were fine.

Göksal became a constant texting buddy for a few weeks. He asked me to send photos and to "massaj" my hair. Nearly three years later, he still likes all my Facebook photos – at least the ones that show my hair.

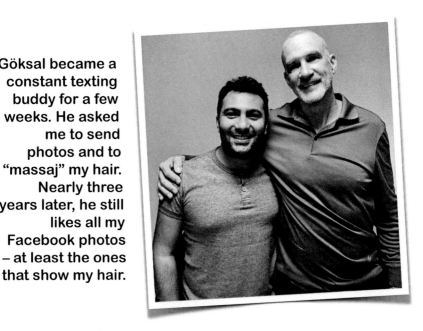

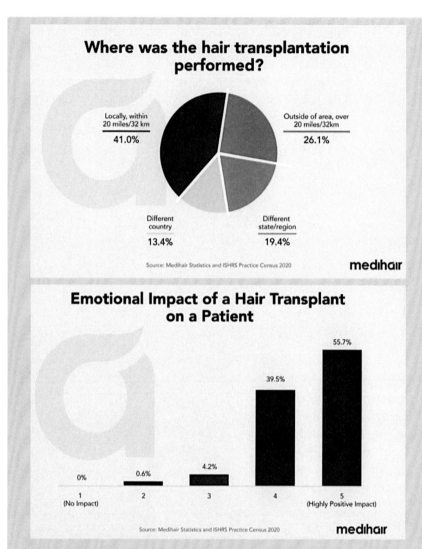

Where was the hair transplantation performed?

Locally, within
20 miles/32 km
41.0%

Outside of area, over
20 miles/32km
26.1%

Different
country
13.4%

Different
state/region
19.4%

Source: Medihair Statistics and ISHRS Practice Census 2020

medihair

Emotional Impact of a Hair Transplant on a Patient

55.7%

39.5%

4.2%

0%

0.6%

1
(No Impact)

2

3

4

5
(Highly Positive Impact)

Source: Medihair Statistics and ISHRS Practice Census 2020

medihair

Medihair's founder **Kilian C. Wisskirchen** began to notice the effects of hair loss on his hair line and started conducting research on the topic. He was overwhelmed with the mass of information and products claiming to prevent hair loss or restore growth. In reality, only a portion of these treatments were scientifically proven, and some of the information was simply incorrect. After extensive research and sorting through the hair loss myths on the internet he decided to build a platform where he could share his knowledge with others. This led to the creation of medihair.com.

10. Going Public With My "New" Hair

With our medical tourism trip nearly complete, we spent one last night in Istanbul before preparing to check out of our hotel. Before leaving for the Istanbul airport, I had made arrangements to meet with a local PR firm owner – part of my business development efforts for my digital company. I wasn't sure what I would look like at that point, the day after the bandages were removed, but I thought slipping in a business meeting would be useful. Çınar Ergin, the head of Aristo Communications, was intrigued enough to agree to a meeting.

A few hours before our afternoon flight back home, I wondered if the meeting was a smart idea with my head in its early recovery period. Çınar's office was in a beautiful older section of the city on İstiklal Street on the European side of the Bosporus. Surrounded by churches, museums, and diplomatic residences, I was so glad I visited that area and it added to my desire to return one day to Istanbul as a regular tourist to visit it and other parts of the ancient city.

As I walked into the front of Çınar's office, I looked on the wall of his reception area and saw a display of their clients. One was an Istanbul facility for hair transplants, so I knew Çınar would recognize my condition and perhaps tease me why I didn't visit his

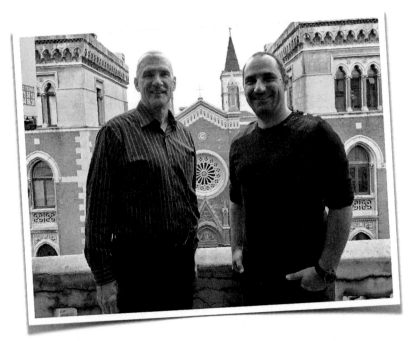

Day 2 post-surgery: My first sales call with Çınar Ergin of Aristo Communications, who hosted coffee and a tour of his cool office on İstiklal Street, downtown Istanbul.

client. Instead, Çınar, whose hair was not much longer than mine, was a wonderful host, offering me coffee, a tour of his office, and agreed to a photo from one of their porches with an inspiring view of the old city. We agreed to stay in touch and I left – with Çınar never bringing up my slightly bloody scalp. I thought perhaps he was merely being kind as he certainly surmised why I was in town. Yet, his unexpected acceptance of my appearance, such as it was, without questions or comments, set the tone for nearly all the other encounters I'd have in the coming two years.

I hurried back to the hotel where Kevin's rental car was at the front door. He was in the lobby and Mike was ... not there. Unfortunately, Mike had contracted my cold and developed a worse case than I had. He was in bed, napping, and when we roused him, he got up, grabbed his bag, and headed out the door. We drove to the new airport, nearly an hour out of town, but worth the drive just to see other parts of Istanbul as well as the impressive approach to the country's aviation investment. My previous trips into Istanbul were through the old airport, which was squeezed into a hilly portion of the city. That always made landings and takeoffs a bit more thrilling and visually stunning.

The new airport was massive in scale and extremely well organized. Yet, as we stepped toward the check-in desk at the terminal, I heard Mike behind me say a curse word – one he doesn't use often. Without turning, I guessed what had happened – he had left his passport in the hotel safe and, in our rushing him to the lobby, didn't grab it before leaving. We were faced with leaving him there to return to the hotel and getting his own flight back. I suggested Kevin call the hotel and hire a taxi to drive Mike's passport the hour to the airport. "Great idea," Kevin said. It worked and Mike was able to hop on our flight just before takeoff.

As we wandered through the cavernous facility waiting for Mike, I noticed what Kevin predicted: other men wearing either telltale post-surgical bandages or beautifully bare, recently transplanted headscapes. Whenever I could catch the eye of a fellow patient, no matter what age they were or if they were from Syria, South Africa, or South America, for that one moment in time at the new Istanbul airport, we were brothers. We were all heading back to re-inject ourselves into our previous lives and to face an uncertain response from our respective coworkers, family, and friends, but each of us had independently come to our own individual conclusions that being bald was not how we saw ourselves in our minds and, after today, was not how anyone was ever going to see us in reality. As I passed them, I'd nod my head and smile slightly and often they'd do the same in return.

Having hair on top of my head for the first time in decades gave me a sense of momentum, of validation – similar to the strength that begins to enter my shoulders and biceps and thighs in the third or fourth week of consistently going to the gym three times a week. In each instance, a glance in the mirror revealed a barely perceptible improvement in my body, but it was there nonetheless.

There's that feeling that things are on the move and all for the better. Where before there might have been that tiny gap of confidence preventing you from being your full self with a full head of hair, now that has been fixed and that little gap is instead filled with a small yet warm, self-affirming buzz. It's a buzz that for years had been missing or, at best, elusive. It was sort of like those moments when you've just crossed the threshold of an early alcohol buzz when, if you just didn't drink anymore, you'd have a nice consistent lift.

With this frosty layer of angel hair glistening atop a previously barren headscape, there isn't a danger that you'll feel too much too soon as with alcohol. You cannot hurry it, but this good feeling is here to stay. No matter how many vitamins you swallow or how much care you give to your tender scalp, you have no choice other than to wait for nature to take its indefatigable and inexorable course of replenishing the top of your head with those long-lost beautiful strands of hair that were so much a part of your youth.

Research says ...

The International Society of Hair Restoration Surgery, a non-profit medical association with more than 1,000 members in 70 countries, published these results from its 2020 Census Results about hair restoration surgical procedures:

– 66% used FUE harvesting, 29.8% used strip harvesting

– 92.5% harvested hair from scalp, 7.5% beard, 2.4% chest, less than 1% from belly, leg and "other"

– 57.2% had one procedure, 33.1% had two, 9.6% three+

– Internationally, 84.2% of patients were male

– 81% transplant between 1000-3000 grafts

– 4% were 20-25 of age, 45.2% were 26-35, 42.2% were 36-45, 8.6% were 46-60, 0% were 61+

– **34.7% cited career/professional reasons for restoration, 37% social/dating**

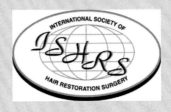

11. Coming Home to Heal

When I got home, I walked in the front door and turned on the hallway chandelier. Jan came down the steps, stepped back and looked at me, now seeing the tiny fuzz of hair all around my head, tinged a slight red from the small amount of blood hugging some of my follicles. Her eyes were electric. She smiled.

"You look cool," she said and hugged me.

" I know," I said. "I almost decided to shave it and stay bald."

"I'm glad you didn't," she said.

"I think I look like Bruce Willis," I said.

"I wouldn't go that far," Jan said. "But you do look cool."

It was early November 2019. I would have preferred to stay home for a few months and let my head recover, but we had a gauntlet of social events to navigate before the spring would bring the sprouting – and the preferred official grand introduction of my crop of permanent hair. I was cognizant that at any moment, all the new hair planted on top of my head could fall out – not to mention the surviving hairs around the side of my head.

With thousands of lifelong neighbors suddenly removed, how would these hairs react to their sudden trauma? My side hair was not in danger of falling out, Göksal has assured me. Yet, with a suddenly thinner forest, would the hairs bend, lie flatter, and break off, depreciating what had been a thick band of my remaining hair?

Within a few days after I returned from Istanbul, I didn't present a very elegant tableau. The hair was tiny and fuzzy. My scalp was clear cut, betraying a soft, overall taint of a glow I called irritated red. There was still some random blood spots, but thanks to the fact that I could begin shampooing my hair 48 hours after my final visit with Göksal, my headscape was beginning to return to normal. Yet it was way too early for my field of follicles to present any semblance of the promised head of hair to come.

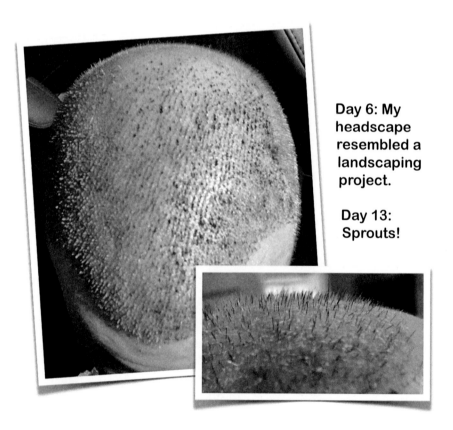

Day 6: My headscape resembled a landscaping project.

Day 13: Sprouts!

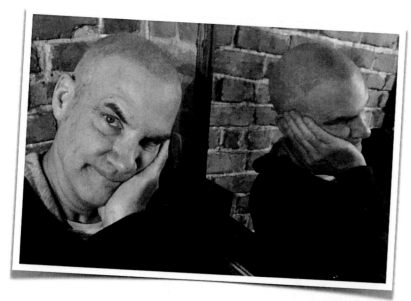

Day 9: When high school classmate Hamp Skelton offered his cool pad in New Orleans' Bywater as a place to hide and heal, I jumped. Göksal insisted on daily photos. I enjoyed my favorite town as a backdrop.

Göksal became a daily fixture in my life through the messaging app WhatsApp. Each morning – afternoon for him – I'd get a text from him asking for an update and requesting that I send him photos. He was pleased with my progress.

When I seemed too optimistic about the prospects of my hair not falling out, he cautioned me to be realistic and to not be disappointed if and when it did disappear. He promised it would return a few weeks later. He also checked to make sure I was taking the vitamins and he also suggested I gently massage my

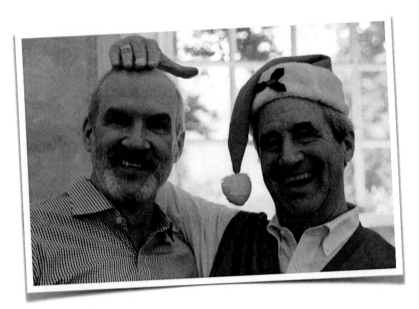

Day 56, Christmas: Brother Jack getting a little too close to those babies just crawling out on my head.

scalp regularly. "Hair likes massaj. Massaj is good," he would text me almost daily in his endearing attempts at English.

Meanwhile, I figured it might be wise to condition my high school buddies to my new look. It started just as I'd planned: at lunch with a dozen of them at a long table at Murphy's, an Atlanta restaurant owned for 40 years by grade-school pal and Irishman Tom Murphy, who had bailed on going with me to Istanbul.

When Tom asked me in front of the group why I'd made the change, I delivered my planned joke, "I asked Jan what she wanted for her 60th birthday and she said, 'Just once before I die I'd like to make love to a man with a full head of hair,' " then paused two beats before delivering my rehearsed punchline.

Instead, Norris Broyles – an architect who grew up on my street, went to the University of Virginia with me, and appears to have never lost one hair despite his dad being bald as a cue-ball for all of our memories – beat me to the punch. He quickly intoned dryly, "Give her my number." That led to a hearty round of laughs from my friends who were then ready to move on to other subjects.

At a social event just a few weeks later, one of two early childhood friends, Ken Smith, seemed keenly interested. His now-deceased dad and all of his four living brothers were severely bald, yet Ken was the outlier in many ways, including his ability to cultivate a thick head of hair. Yet even Ken, in the past two or three years, had begun to shed more follicles than he'd expected. Jan and I walked into the home where the wine tasting was being hosted and quickly stepped toward the second or third room, near the bar.

At the end of this main room were two steps to an upper level of the room that transitioned to a higher outside deck. Ken stood above me on the upper level next to his brother Bill, who was the youngest in his family and perhaps, like me, the most bald of all his brothers. They looked over my scalp like two farmers leaning over a fence, eyeing a neighbor's just-planted field. They didn't say anything – they just looked at my scalp – for more than an awkward moment. I tried to enlist Bill's interest in the investment I had just made, but neither he nor Ken said much at all.

Later that evening, Ken shared how his wife Caryl poked him, suggesting he might consider going to Istanbul to get a few hairs moved to the frontal region of his head from where many of his hairs had recently departed. Before I could ask if Ken was interested in going to Istanbul, my other early childhood friend, Mike Egan, wandered over. Mike, who was also just starting to thin in what had otherwise always been an enviable head of northern European hair, lifted his glass of scotch and proposed a toast to the "last time we'll ever see Schro without hair."

A few Wednesdays later, I stepped off a flight returning from a Boston business trip at nearly the exact same moment Jan exited a flight from Louisiana, where she had attended a travel writers conference. Walking down the concourse at the Atlanta airport, towards the "plane train" to return to our car, Jan confided a few attendees had previously attended a New Orleans conference that was named an early hot spot of a virus that was rapidly spreading across America, COVID-19.

Two days later – four months after I had returned from Istanbul and just as 5,000 hairs were beginning to poke out from their new homes to show off – Jan and I locked our front door and began sheltering inside the confines of our four walls for much of the next year. The rest of the globe was doing the same.

This lockdown wasn't at all configured into my rollout plan and its several contingencies. I had timed my trip and the hoped-for growth of my new hair to be revealed at a series of April events. These included annual galas for a few business groups of which I was a member as well as a college fraternity reunion in Charlottesville, Virginia, and a three-day public relations conference of 150 longtime business associates that would be hosted in Puerto Vallarta, Mexico.

During the months leading up to my Istanbul trip, I had envisioned my Great Reveal – walking first into commercial real estate networking groups, rendering my clients, mostly conservative Republican developers, speechless. I'd then planned to point to my new hair, saying, "My doctor diagnosed it as the crowning proof of global warming." I had imagined walking into the PR Counselors Academy conference of which I was a sponsor and suddenly having the young agency owners who might have resisted my sales pitches before be more attracted to listening to my offerings. As for my April fraternity reunion, I had fully expected a rousing series of ribbings – and head rubbings – from several classes of brothers who would stand in marvel of my new look and give me mounds of grief about it.

Instead of my plan – attending this gauntlet of events in which I was a well-known and long-standing member and telling and hearing well-timed jokes about my hair – my new field of tender follicles started to grow in just as the 2020 worldwide pandemic fell out. Jan and I were left to marvel at my hair all by ourselves.

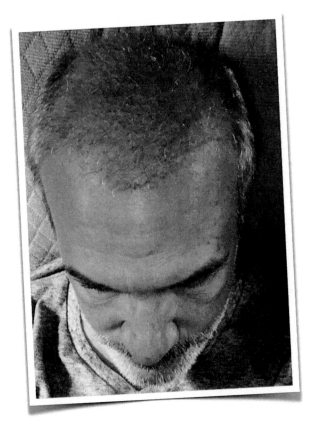

Day 90: My landscaping project grew into a forest! Well, maybe for an optimist like me.

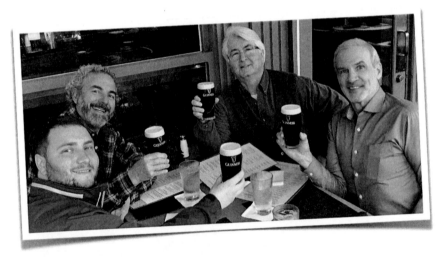

Day 137, St. Patrick's Day: Our last Guinness and the last lunch served at Murphy's before the shutdown, with Graham Massell, Steve Massell, and Tom Murphy. As for my hair, I was feeling the luck of the Irish.

12. Watch Out For Those Freckles

P artly to satisfy Göksal's request for photographic updates and partly because I thought one day I'd satisfy my friends' curiosity by chronicling my journey in a blog or perhaps a magazine article, I began taking photos of my progress. Each day or two of the shutdown, I would stand in front of my bathroom mirror and shoot selfies. One day, I began comparing my look to photos I had taken just a few days prior. Up above, I didn't see a lot of growth at first, but I was glad to see the redness start to dissipate. I was also pleased that my hairs never fell out in their post-traumatic move to my crown as predicted. I attributed this anomaly to my having eaten seed bars with millet for years before my surgery and after.

Just before closing my most recent photo, I happened to notice a spot on my right shoulder that I didn't remember. I went back and compared it with previous photos from that month and I noticed that the spot not only had appeared in only the most recent photos, but that it was darkening quickly with each passing day and that the spot was not round or symmetrical like my other freckles and moles. I began to worry that I might be developing a melanoma.

I remembered that my brother Mike had recently told our siblings that he had a melanoma spot removed from his shoulder. I

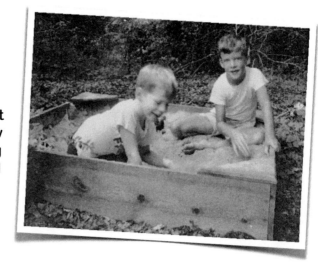

Age 6: What did we know about playing in the sun all day long? Ken Smith and me in the sandbox.

also knew that Jan's father had died of cancer just two years before and that it had begun with a diagnosis of melanoma. When I told Jan about my spot and showed her the photos, she urged me to call my primary physician, Dr. Alan Perry, immediately. I called Dr. Perry the next day. While he couldn't see me in person due to the pandemic protocols, he asked me to upload the photos to the healthcare portal. He looked over the photos and called me back.

Dr. Perry is a jovial general practitioner whom Jan and I always loved seeing for our healthcare visits. He maintains a caring, professional tone with a casual delivery sometimes coupled with a clever quip that never fails to put us at ease. In this phone call, he was not jovial or clever. He was serious when he said, "It may not be the best time for this to be happening, given the shutdown, but I think you should set up an appointment with the dermatologist and have them do a biopsy just to be safe. Don't delay."

At my dermatological appointment, everyone in their office was careful to wear masks, check my temperature, and maintain distance except when they had to look at my shoulder and slice off the spot to send to the lab for diagnosis. The dermatologist was, like Dr. Perry, extremely personable and likable. She took a special interest in my scalp. I told her of my recent hair transplant surgery in Istanbul and, when I told her I might write a magazine article about my experience, she gave me her cell phone number and asked that I call her when it was finished because she would like to know more about the process and pass it on to a few bald men she thought might be interested.

I was of that Caucasian generation that believed "brown is beautiful" and we spent way too much time in the sun as children without proper sunscreen. While my brother Mike had a more sensitive complexion, my brother Jack was very swarthy and tanned easily and deeply. I was somewhere in between. I actually remember my worst sunburn as a child when our class went on a field trip to Callaway Gardens resort in Georgia. I was busy in the sand building a sand castle with Ken Smith and others and I recall our teacher asking me several times if I wanted to apply "sun tan lotion," which back then I thought accelerated rather than prevented the sun's dangerous rays. I was adamant in my refusal of the lotion, as a young boy often is in the face of an authoritative suggestion. The next day, I woke up with a horrific sunburn on my shoulders and back and missed at least one day of school as I screamed in pain in my bed. That no doubt was the precursor of this very shoulder spot we were concerned with in my early sixties.

After the dermatologist cut the sample off my shoulder, as an aside, I mentioned another spot that had troubled me since it appeared at the very tip of my nose after I returned from a conference in Scottsdale, Arizona. The May 1984 conference was extremely hot, above 100 degrees – but it was "a dry heat," as Arizonans are wont to say. I had socialized by the pool and played golf on the course at the Camelback Inn, where the conference was hosted.

Within days of my return to Greenville, South Carolina, where we then lived, I told my first wife about my spot and she too urged me to go to a dermatologist as the tiny spot was growing darker. After studying it closely, I remember the doctor saying the spot could be pre-cancerous and it would be smart to go ahead and remove it right away to ensure it didn't evolve into something

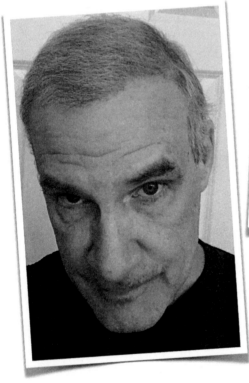
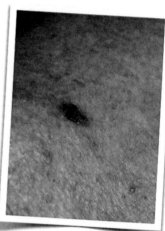

Day 151: Hair's looking fine, but my attention turns again to the spot on the nose ... and a new one I notice on my shoulder on Day 157.

more serious later. I agreed, but was horrified when he pulled out an instrument that was basically a small drill with a curled tip that I compared to a wine opener. As he drilled the shaft into the end of my nose, I kept thinking that surely there had to be better medical procedures for such skin removal than a modified wine opener. It took years for that scar to return to normal and I made a vow to make sure I only visited dermatologists in the future who had better equipment.

Through those years, I had occasionally visited dermatologists as part of my healthcare routine – perhaps once a decade for other matters such as athlete's foot or removal of spots or warts. Each visit, whether it was in Greenville, Charlotte, or Atlanta, I had casually mentioned that the spot on my nose had returned and I told each of the doctors of the wine opener tool and they winced as I had. They would look at my nose and each one came to the same conclusion: "It looks like a simple freckle and there probably isn't anything to worry about at the moment."

That was the same response I received from my current dermatologist. While she and her staff were appropriately concerned about the shoulder, they were not so much interested in the spot on my nose. A few days later, their office assistant called and said the shoulder spot had indeed been analyzed as a melanoma and they immediately referred me to a skin surgeon, Dr. Katarina Nalovic, who specialized in an advanced procedure called Mohs Surgery.

I was amazed by what I called the choreography of Dr. Nalovic's office. I counted up to 10 different healthcare professionals on her team who stopped by briefly to see me in my chair, touch my shoulder, ask different questions, and answer any of mine. When Dr. Nalovic appeared, I told her how impressed I was by her team and the number of touches I received. She and I had a similar sense of humor and we bonded quickly over a few controversial topics.

As she performed the procedure – which involved slicing off successive microscopic layers from my shoulder, studying them under a special scope to detect cancerous cells, and then, if needed, to remove and analyze deeper layers – I also mentioned the spot on my nose. She took additional time to study it and, even though it wasn't within the scope of my referral to her, she was very adamant in her instruction:

"I want you to march right back into that dermatologist's office as soon as possible and demand that they biopsy this spot on your nose. Don't let them dismiss it."

When I did return to the dermatologist's office, I thought I detected a slight annoyance on the team's part that I had gone over their heads for a second opinion and was now returning with a mandate to change their protocol. Nevertheless, they obliged, quickly took a significant slice off the end of my nose, and sent it to the lab for analysis. Two days later, they called and said it was, in fact, melanoma and set me up with another Mohs Surgery appointment with Dr. Nalovic.

This time I was concerned for two reasons. I had gone back and looked at photographs through the years and I noticed the spot had changed colors, darker and lighter. I thought I had sensed a change over time, but since numerous dermatologists had discounted what looked like a freckle, I just assumed it, like some other freckles, changed shades with the seasons and varying exposure to the sun.

Secondly, while Dr. Nalovic was pleased she only had to remove a minimal number of layers of skin before she was satisfied she had gotten all concerning cells on my shoulder, the stitching together of the wound resulted in a significant area that needed a lot of time to heal. I could only imagine what such a similar wound and resultant scarring would occur on a more sensitive – and prominent – area of my headscape such as my nose.

Dr. Nalovic and team did in fact remove and analyze several layers on my nose. When they were satisfied that they had removed enough to extract all the concerning cancer cells, her team pulled several flaps from different quadrants of my nose back over the tip and stitched them together. My nose looked like railroad tracks had been built over its contours.

Ever since my shoulder and nose melanomas, my dermatologist's team has persistently scheduled semi-annual full-body screenings during which they scrutinize and make a note of every spot on my body. Ironically, one year later, one skin flap that Dr. Nalovic had

Day 233: My siblings always said I looked like our great-grandfather, Jack Spalding, co-founder of King & Spalding law firm. On Father's Day, I took photos of my dad and his dad, William, son-in-law of Jack, who's in the portrait.

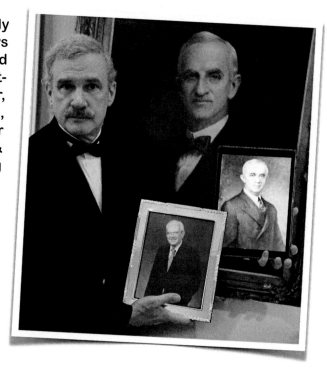

pulled from the side of my nose and stitched over the tip developed a darkening spot on the same spot as the original. My dermatologist was quick to analyze that it wasn't melanoma, yet was cautious enough to freeze it with liquid nitrogen twice in a year to discourage it from developing into cancer. I have confidence they won't miss future developing melanomas.

When I got home and showed Jan the photograph of my stitched-up nose that had since been covered with bandages, she said, "Oh my gosh. That's worse than I thought. With those big black stitches, you look like you have a Franken-nose." A few days later, when I hosted a Zoom call with my brothers and sisters Van, and Suzanne, to celebrate a cluster of birthdays, I shared the photograph with them. They were as shocked as Jan had been. It was really ugly.

My brother-in-law Joe, who's in his 80s and not quite up-to-speed on Zoom, kept leaning into the laptop screen and interrupting our conversation. He assumed he was making private comments to my sister. "Suzanne," he kept saying. "Chris looks like an entirely different person with that hair." He said nothing about my nose.

I wrestled with several thoughts. First, I was thankful to have spotted the melanoma early and to have gotten such good medical care. Secondly, I was annoyed different dermatologists through the decades had concluded the spot on my nose was not anything to worry about. Third, I was thankful I had mentioned the spot to Dr. Nalovic during my shoulder surgery and that she was adamant I demand a biopsy.

I also realized that my decision to invest in hair transplantation – which could and perhaps should be viewed as a self-absorbed, vain effort to reverse God-ordained male pattern baldness – had in an unintended, circuitous way prevented a metastasization of melanoma from my shoulder to other organs in my body.

In short, my decision to transplant my hair may have saved my life.

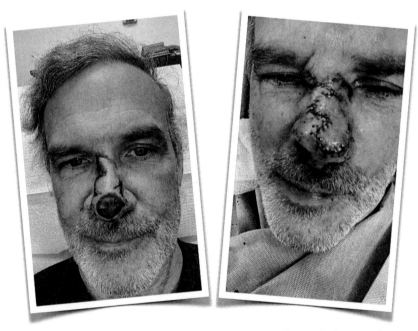

Day 300: The dermatologist took a slice at the end and the surgeon went deeper, sewing my nose up with what seemed like railroad tracks over my face.

13. Time For The Table

J ust prior to my 1992 marital separation from my first wife, I began a spiritual journey that led to my joining the Friday Morning Men's Fellowship, a weekly Bible study run by Leadership Ministries. Its founder and leader, Chris White, who is significantly bald, also leads my small group of eight to 10 men who meet for an hour after our larger-session sermon.

Occasionally, as Chris gathers our "table" for coffee, doughnuts, and instruction, our table-mate Bob Voyles, who maintains and sometimes strokes a thick crop of youthful California-surfer-like blond hair, needles Chris about his bald head "shining too brightly for us to see the others." Chris usually responds quickly, saying, "Grass doesn't grow on a busy street."

I've heard Chris, a learned Bible scholar whose ministry has expanded to several Southeastern cities, quote Luke 14:11: "For all those who exalt themselves will be humbled, and those who humble themselves will be exalted." As I now gazed in the mirror at my incoming hair and below at the railroad crossing that covered my nose, I couldn't help but smile at how God humbled me with my front-and-center facial surgery immediately following my self-exalting effort to reorganize my hair.

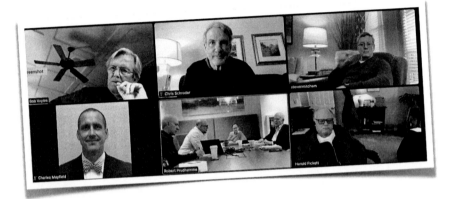

**Hybrid Friday Morning Men's Fellowship meeting.
Bob Voyles taking notes, top left; Chris White lighting up
the table as always, bottom center, right side of table.**

When I joined the Friday morning Zoom call a couple of days after my nose surgery, I disabled Zoom's video feature, joining with audio only. When Bob asked why I wasn't on video, I said it was because my nose looked like Karl Malden's in Elia Kazan's 1954 film *On The Waterfront*. Bob and my table-mates laughed loudly.

Before agreeing to my hair transplants, I had actually wrestled with the fact that my male pattern baldness was apparently God's plan for me and programmed into my personal genetic algorithm. I wasn't sure it was wise to "mess with Mother Nature" and that I should instead accept my fate and quote, as many bald men are wont to: "God made few perfect heads … the others he covered with hair."

There was also the fact there are countless unsuccessful examples of attempts by men through the decades to escape their baldness with hair plugs, strips, and even transplants. Also, there might be a reason why my mother, society in general, and even I have such a visceral aversion to toupees, comb-overs, and other attempts to hide baldness. I had grown comfortable with Kevin's championing of hair transplantation through the years and was reassured by the previous patients of Göksal who'd reported how pleased they were with their results. I also gained confidence due to the evolution of Jan and her encouragement to consider so dramatically changing my appearance. If there is anyone on the planet more skeptical, practical, and analytical than Jan, I've yet to meet them, much less marry them.

Plus, there were my incredulous friends, a very select few of whom I had consulted before agreeing to the surgery. Representative of their views was David Martin, a nurse who's built two vascular surgery startups and who sports a healthy head of gray-flecked brown hair. Before committing to the trip, I shared my plans with him. His prognosis: "I predict this won't end well."

Tom "TC" Calk – a buddy since 7th grade who just retired from a stellar 40-year career as a pediatrician, allowing him to begin pulling his fully intact brown hair into a retirement-induced pony tail – was also squarely planted in the skeptics camp. When I confided in him my plans to go to Istanbul for the procedure, he cautioned, "From a medical point of view, I do not endorse this. Too many things can go wrong – and probably will."

I had not joined my Friday morning table in person since before my November return from Istanbul, partly due to my strategy to not show my scars to familiar groups – outside immediate family and buddies – before my hair had a chance to grow in. I was also still reticent to appear in large groups since COVID-19 was still pushing its deadly tentacles around the world. Mostly my absence was due to travel. I had extended my frenetic out-of-town business travel schedule into the first part of 2020 and this often caused me to be out of town on Friday mornings.

Yet, despite the fact that, beginning in April 2020, my image had been projected via Zoom in a small video square onto computer screens of the eight to 12 men in my Friday morning men's group, not one of them had said word one about the growing fuzz appearing on the top of my head. Surely, they had seen a change in my appearance, so why had they chosen not to say anything at all? It seemed as unnatural as my sudden hair growth.

This failure to address the changes atop the very dome from which my table-mates sat across for nearly three decades was puzzling to me. What were they thinking? Could they not see my hair in their Zoom windows? Or did they see my new young follicle cultivation and not know what to say? Or were they questioning their own memory of my previous baldness? Or worse, did they not even notice I was now cultivating a fresh crop of hair? Were my years of feeling angst and inadequate about my receding hairline wasted? Was I the only one who rated my dome as my most prominent physical feature? Was my globe-trotting $7,000 investment to change my appearance mere folly? Was my self-doubt based on my ever-encroaching baldness a battle that raged only in my cranial cavity a millimeter or two below the shiny skin on which I had been so focused?

As it turned out, my table-mates' reaction – or non-reaction – wasn't an anomaly. It was the beginning of what I found to be a puzzling and completely unexpected reaction by nearly everyone I encountered for the next year or two.

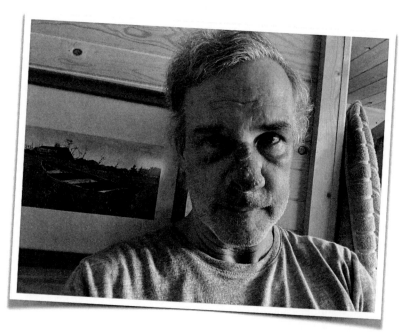

Day 304: Still a work in progress, but definitely feeling positive about the talents of Göksal and Dr. Nalovic. Considering career as doppelgänger for Karl Malden.

Samson and Delilah ...

Then she said to him, "How can you say, 'I love you,' when you won't confide in me? This is the third time you have made a fool of me and haven't told me the secret of your great strength."

With such nagging she prodded him day after day until he was sick to death of it. So he told her everything. "No razor has ever been used on my head," he said, "because I have been a Nazirite dedicated to God from my mother's womb. If my head were shaved, my strength would leave me, and I would become as weak as any other man."

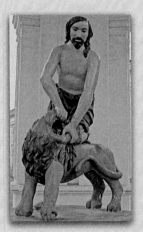

The Fountain of Samson, Kiev, Ukraine

When Delilah saw that he had told her everything, she sent word to the rulers of the Philistines, "Come back once more; he has told me everything." So the rulers of the Philistines returned with the silver in their hands. After putting him to sleep on her lap, she called for someone to shave off the seven braids of his hair, and so began to subdue him. And his strength left him.

Then she called, "Samson, the Philistines are upon you!" He awoke from his sleep and thought, "I'll go out as before and shake myself free." But he did not know that the Lord had left him. Then the Philistines seized him, gouged out his eyes and took him down to Gaza. Binding him with bronze shackles, they set him to grinding grain in the prison.

But the hair on his head began to grow again after it had been shaved.

– Judges 16: 15-22, NIV

14. Breaking Out Of The Lockdown

As the first weeks of the pandemic extended into months, Jan and I, like all of the world, made adjustments to our lives. Jan is a travel writer. Once or twice a month, she would fly out to a new destination where she'd be wined, dined, and shuttled to local notable venues so she could present her experiences to the 500,000 readers of our newsletter, The Travel 100. In the prior four years, I'd fly out nearly every week, calling on PR firm owners, urging them to launch newsletters and websites populated with our curated 100-word-story formula. Suddenly, in mid-March 2020, our travel schedules came to a stop. Like billions of others around the globe, Jan and I adjusted to what we discovered was a more sane and sustainable lifestyle confined to the footprint of our own homes. We cooked, read, cleaned our closets, took long walks, and offset our growing isolation with increasing numbers of Zoom calls. Video calls proved adequate – but not ideal to spurring reactions to a new product, service or, as in my case, a new appearance.

One day, Jan had an idea to soften our seclusion. She sent an email to owners of the 24 townhomes on our circle, suggesting we meet that Friday at 5:30 p.m. for a socially distanced cocktail party. Surely, I thought, this in-person community gathering would lead to at least one of our neighbors commenting on my changed appearance. As we dragged our folding chairs and custom cocktails onto our street, everyone was elated to see familiar humanity. Nearly two dozen neighbors chose to join in the springtime gatherings and swap stories of lifestyle adjustments, family news, and most important, which nearby restaurants we'd each discovered provided excellent takeout or, thanks to recent changes in local legislation, alcoholic drinks to go. As Jan and I hosted the neighbors clustering around our driveway, I waited for comments on my new hair. Instead, there was silence on that matter.

One neighbor, who we all called Coach, approached me and finally said something. Coach, who was nearly as bald on top as I once had been, looked all around my head, then said, "Chris … tell me … you used to have a beard, right? Did you shave it off?"

"No, Coach," I said. "I haven't had a beard in quite a while."

He seemed puzzled, but not nearly as much as I was by his confusion. I couldn't help but smile as he kept looking at me, unable to detect the difference in my appearance since he last saw me.

The awkward avoidance of what I thought was the elephant in the room or, in this case, street, reminded me of a four-day jury on which I'd served more than a decade before to adjudicate a criminal rape case. As members of our 12-person jury spent time cloistered in seclusion while the judge and lawyers debated motions, not one person in our midst addressed an obvious situation – that one of our jurors was Kevin Millwood, an Atlanta Braves pitcher who had, just weeks before in his first postseason appearance, become the first person to pitch a one-hitter in a division playoff. This spectacular win occurred against the Houston Astros in the National League Division Series. He lasted slightly more than two innings in a World Series loss to the New York Yankees a few weeks later.

Everyone on the jury assumed everyone else on the jury had recently spent hours watching him pitch and recognized him immediately when he was named to our panel. Everyone, except one woman, who sat next to him before we were about to begin deliberations. The room fell silent as we listened to her engage him in small chitchat. For three days, we had all respected his privacy and none of us had the courage to break the ice about his celebrity. Kevin and the woman were chatting when she asked him if he had finished his Christmas shopping. Kevin, a handsome, humble man from Gaston County, North Carolina, who'd nicely talked with her at length, answered her politely.

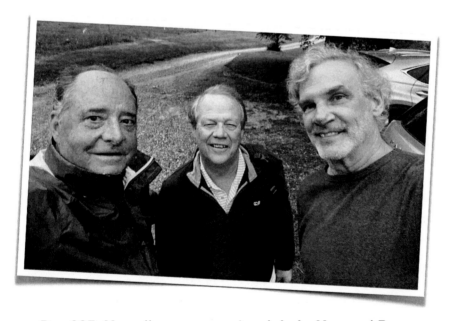

Day 327: My college roommates, Irénée May and Beau Grenier, at our spontaneous 2020 Lake James, NC, reunion.

"Yes, ma'am, I've done most of my shopping."

"Really," she asked? "Most men wait until the last minute. Where did you do your shopping?"

"Well," Kevin answered slowly in his smart southern drawl. "I was able to do all my shopping in the clubhouse store."

"Clubhouse store?" she asked. "What is the clubhouse store?"

"Well, ma'am," he said. "It's the Braves clubhouse store. The Atlanta Braves store."

The rest of us were all quiet, watching this unfold as if we were witnessing a slow-motion car wreck at a country crossroads. The woman slowly turned, looked him over and gasped.

"Are you that World Series pitcher?"

"Yes'm," Kevin mumbled to her quietly. "Yes ma'am. I'm Kevin Millwood. It's nice to make your acquaintance."

She squealed in delight.

"Oh, my word," she yelled. "I'm so sorry I didn't recognize you. Would you sign an autograph for my grandson? He'd kill me if I told him I served on the jury with you and didn't get your autograph."

"Sure, ma'am," he said. "I'd be happy to."

The room erupted in relief, laughter, and delight as if peace had just been restored between two good friends who were on the edge of a fist fight and had instead settled the score and hugged. The two bailiffs who had been with us constantly that week as well as all the jurors grabbed paper and pens and got in line for Kevin to sign multiple autographs for each of us to give as Christmas presents.

Each week, our neighbors would pull out their chairs on Friday afternoon and share stories of pandemic survival and get to know each other in ways we never had before COVID-19, when we'd merely wave at each other before driving into our separate garages.

Finally, one Friday afternoon, when the wind was blowing and my hair, which I had not trimmed since Göksal's team had cut it to near skinhead length six months before, was beginning to look a little unruly. A couple who had just moved into the neighborhood joined our party and introduced themselves to each of us and edged a little closer than the prescribed six-foot distance we had been observing during our weekly outings.

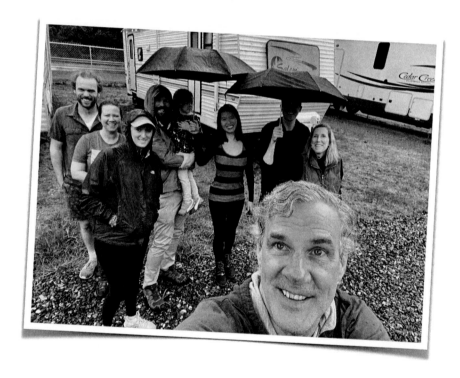

Day 345: Nearly a year later, not even a NC storm could dampen our spirits. Checking out the camper: Alex Fritz, Sally, Amanda, Thomas and Annie Schroder, Holly Yan, Chris Butsch and Jan.

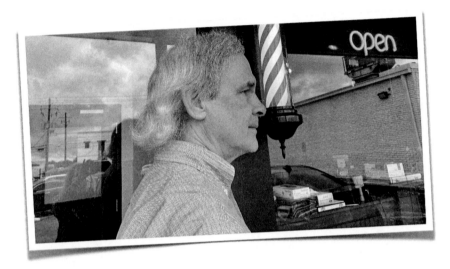

**Day 365: I held out exactly one year for my first haircut.
Jan said I had already entered "crazy old man" territory.**

The husband was extremely bald and seemed intrigued by my hair. "So I guess you haven't had a chance to go to a barber during the lockdown?" the new neighbor asked me.

"No, I have decided I would go an entire year without a haircut since I had my surgery," I told him. All the other neighbors' side conversations fell silent and they watched and listened to our discussion.

"Oh, sorry," he said. "I didn't know you had surgery. What kind of surgery?"

"Well," I said, trying to simulate Kevin Millwood's soft response. "I had hair transplant surgery six months ago. If you had met me then, I'd have been as bald as a cue ball." I pulled out my iPhone and showed him the photo of me reading to my granddaughter Annie.

The new neighbor was taken aback and stepped closer to look at my scalp. All the rest of the neighbors erupted in giggles and pulled their chairs a little closer. He thought he had made a faux pas, when I thought he had merely popped a tightening balloon. For the next 30 minutes, Jan and I told the story of how and why I had gone to Istanbul. Some shared stories of friends or children who were bald and wondered aloud if they should send them by to see Kevin the barber whose shop was merely two blocks south of our circle.

A few days later, Jan and I were on a neighborhood walk when we passed the house of our neighbor who, though I'd never asked him, I was quite confident had invested in hair plugs years before that he now kept covered with ball caps. We talked with him about his most recent pet peeve, neighbors and landscapers who "polluted" our tree-filled hills with the loud, nerve-racking roars of gas-fueled leaf blowers. When we bid adieu and began walking down the street, he yelled back as we were 200 feet past.

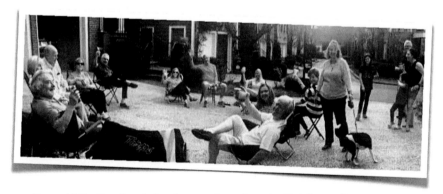

Day 497: Springlake Lane Pandemic Friday afternoons.

"Chris," he hollered. "I meant to ask you. Did you get LASIK eye surgery?"

"What?" I yelled back, confused but also entertained. "No, why do you ask?"

"You look different," he said. "You look younger. I thought it was LASIK surgery."

Jan and I laughed and shook our heads as we kept walking – amazed that a friend, who we assumed was sensitive about his own early-generation hair implants and who should be keenly aware of the change well above my eyes, didn't have a clue.

And so it went.

15. For Your Viewing Pleasure

When my University of Virginia fraternity canceled our April 2020 celebration of the 160th anniversary of the chapter's founding, I emailed the dozen members of my class and suggested a Zoom reunion instead. All quickly agreed. It had been five years since I had seen half of my classmates and more than 40 years since I had seen a few of them. As the hour approached for my appointed hosting of the video session, I carefully brushed and fluffed by hair. I positioned the USB camera and lighting just perfect so it would highlight my new locks.

At 6:30 p.m., I took a sip of my gin and tonic and assumed my classmates were sipping their cocktails, beers, or wine at the same time we clicked through and saw other for the first time in years. The small talk quickly turned into longer questions about one brother's career change, another's move to Oregon, and another's recent birth of a grandchild. We told old stories, just as if we were standing on the porch at old St. Anthony Hall in Charlottesville. As the end of the hour approached, some dropped off to go to dinner, while others lingered to catch up further. As the last one signed off, I walked upstairs to report to Jan how the call went.

"What did they say about your hair?" she asked.

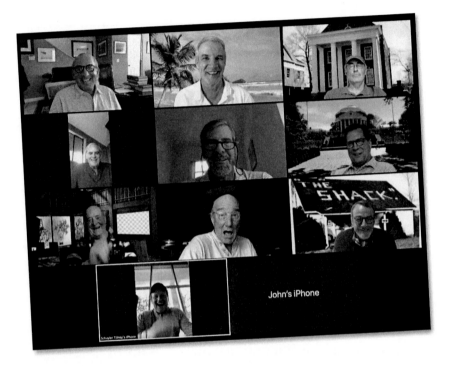

We couldn't celebrate the 160th anniversary of our UVA fraternity in person, so I organized Zoom class reunions. Hank West, of "Two-Mile Island" fame, is center 3rd row.

"No one said a word," I replied.

"What?" she responded. We both shook our heads in amazement. "I expected a boatload of abuse," I said. None was in the cards.

When I joined in on a PR Zoom "cocktail reception" that served as a replacement for our canceled April conference in Puerto Vallarta, people asked how things were going with The 100 Companies or life in Atlanta, but not one soul mentioned my hair.

The same thing occurred when we had socially distanced dinners at outdoor restaurants or in parks with friends. Jan and I would laugh as we left not knowing how anyone would fail to mention my hair. They would almost always make other flattering comments that they'd never made before. The comments rotated between: "Chris, you really look great" or "have you lost weight?" or most frequently: "Chris, you look so young!" We could tell they were wrestling with contributing factors, but no one was asking about my hair, which was starting to grow longer and reach over my forehead and temple.

Through Summer 2020, if we weren't staying home, jumping on Zoom calls or reading books to my granddaughter on FaceTime, the only trips we felt safe making were to Lake James, North Carolina, where two years before I'd bought seven acres of woods and lakefront and added a classic wood-plank dock with proceeds of my PR firm sale. It was a perfect place for my family to have fun during the pandemic with minimal interactions with others.

Coincidentally, in late September, one of my college roommates, Irénée May, who lived in Connecticut, called seeking advice for places to visit in Western North Carolina. He mainly wanted to know where he and his wife Judy could drive and park an RV they had rented for the upcoming week. Irénée was not aware of my recent lake lot purchase so we laughed as I brought him up to speed, marveled at the coincidence, and I offered my dock as a place we could visit.

I then called our third college roommate, Beau Grenier, and his wife Joy, who lived in Birmingham and, amazingly, they accepted the last-minute invitation to join us just a few days later. I had seen Beau and Irénée on Zoom during our fraternity calls, but I was certain they'd have to say something if we were together in person. By this time, I had gone nearly a year without a trim and my hair was getting relatively long. I liked it, but Jan thought I was bordering on "crazy old man" look.

When we all saw each other in person for the first time, Beau was the first to break the ice: "Schro, what is up with your hair?" We all laughed and I told them the story and asked him why he never said anything on our Zoom calls.

"I saw it on Zoom, but I just didn't know what to say," he said.

There had been a few exceptions to an otherwise wall of silence and confusion.

One day, I was wearing a mandated mask at Costco when I renewed my annual membership card. The woman behind the counter looked at my old card with a small image of me in the corner. She looked at the stored image in her computer and then she looked at me again.

"Mr. Schroder, it looks like we need to take a new photograph," she said, laughing. "I love your hair."

I told her she was one of the first to say anything in the year since surgery.

"It's pretty obvious," she said. "You look a lot younger."

"Thank you for saying something," I said. "It's apparently not obvious to everyone else."

When I made a cameo appearance on two of Jan's Zoom calls, we did get two of our handful of reactions in the entire year. In her call with high school classmates, Elizabeth Spalding, who's also my cousin and whose nickname is "Fuzz," took one look at me and said, "Where'd you get the new 'doo?" In the other call, Jan's college suite mate, Patti Lyman, quickly said, "Love the new hair!"

"Thank you for mentioning it," I said. "We had dinner with Beth and Ray (Abbott, who were also on Jan's college suite mate call) in January and we sat there across the table the entire night and they never said a thing!"

Beth and Ray nodded their heads. "We knew something was going on, but we weren't quite sure what," Ray said.

Other than that, maybe two or three people in the course of the year said anything whatsoever. I purposely did not bring it up.

Finally it was approaching September 2021 and time to attend the first in-person annual conference of the Public Relations Society of America's Counselors Academy in two and a half years. Due to pandemic, it had been postponed twice. Seventy people were registered, which was lower than the before-pandemic attendance of 120 to 150 PR firm owners, but there were many reasons to attend.

It was hosted in Nashville, a fun town that's a beautiful four-hour drive away. And though it was a small conference, all the cool kids

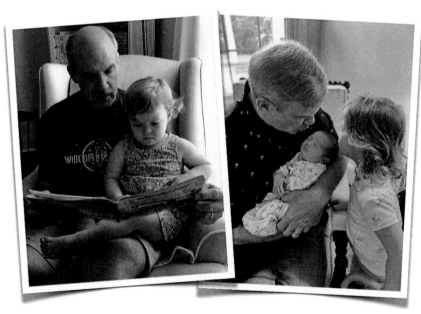

**My go-to, before-and-after photos:
reading to Annie in 2019, loving on her sister Eliza in 2021.**

were going. I had first attended CA as a peer, as a fellow independent agency owner. A few years later, when many friends among the CA attendees signed on to be the first members of my new digital publishing company The 100 Companies, they became clients. In 2017, after Wilbert acquired my agency, allowing me to concentrate on The 100 Companies, I transitioned to not only being a service provider and vendor to CA attendees, but also a sponsor of the conference. Also, as happens, many CA attendees had become close friends over the dozen years I'd been going and I had missed seeing them during the shutdown.

Nearly 75% of PR firm practitioners are women. Men dominate the ranks of upper management in the larger firms, but much of the growth in the industry occurs through the launch of small firms owned predominantly by women in their thirties or forties. In the early years of The 100 Companies, these young female PR firm owners were the most likely prospects for becoming our members.

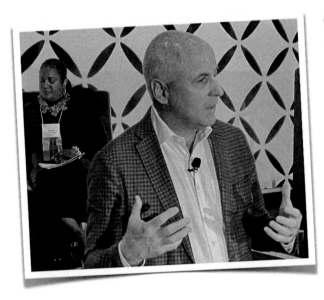

Glen Jackson, leader of Jackson Spalding and a shining exception to the "great hair" CEO rule. He was introduced by another agency owner, Alexis Davis Smith, background.

I'm the primary salesperson for my company and, as you may remember, part of my thinking in investing in hair transplants was to change these women's first impressions of me when I walked into their offices from "old and bald," to just "old." This conference was a chance to test out my new theory, trot out the new hair, and see if my sales success did in fact increase.

Another attraction was that the keynote speaker for the Nashville conference was a colleague and mentor. Glen Jackson co-founded the Jackson Spalding firm with my cousin Bo Spalding two decades ago and quickly grew it to the largest independent firm in Atlanta. They are both very kind, humble, generous men who not only gave me guidance and occasionally referred a client, they allowed my firm to sublease spare office space within theirs during the 2009 Great Recession.

Bo is blessed with a handsome head of thick wavy hair. Glen, a decade or so younger than Bo or me, is follicly challenged. As puerile as it now seems, occasionally when I've stood next to Glen, I'd think that, even though his agency was far more successful and profitable than mine would ever be, at least I had a little more hair than he did. More often, I've stood next to Glen in awe not only of his success and ability to cultivate some of the largest clients in Atlanta and to nurture an enviable team, but also that he's one of the only bald men to run a large agency in America. It seems most of the men who run PR firms in America have "great hair." The same goes for TV news anchors or presidential candidates.

Glen is a deep thinker and he and I have talked about personal, business, and spiritual subjects over breakfasts, but we've never talked about being bald. Men don't do that. We suffer whatever shame we do feel in solitary. The closest we ever get to broaching the subject is speaking an encoded phrase such as: "We have the same barber." Yet I bet Glen was as sad to lose his hair as I was to lose mine. Here, in Nashville, I was curious to see whether he might even notice I was no longer a member of his hair club.

At the opening cocktail reception at the stunning new National Museum of African-American Music, I was excited to see all my friends after a long absence. There were lots of hugs and I took photos of almost everyone in the room to include in our newsletter's slide show. Several people remarked how young I looked. No one at the cocktail party or the small group dinners afterwards mentioned my hair.

The next morning, I spent a few minutes with Glen before and after his keynote speech, taking photos of him on stage and speaking with attendees. We also had a few minutes to catch up alone. I gave him a custom 100-branded mask, which he put on before he left the conference. As we shook hands and said farewell, Glen said, "Good to see you. You look good."

That night at dine-arounds, a dozen of us gathered at a Mexican restaurant. I sat at the corner of the table with Chuck Norman, a Cary, North Carolina, PR firm owner who'd been a good friend and member of The 100 Companies for years. Before dinner, he spotted a large bottle of fine tequila behind the bar and a few at our end of the table shared the final shots in the bottle. Chuck, who has a good head of hair but always keeps it cut relatively short, was occasionally glancing at me and at the top of my head.

Midway through dinner, as the tequila was starting to work its magic, a woman across the table was telling us about her firm and how her new diet helped her shed 80 pounds during the lockdown. She finally asked about my company. Chuck seconded her question, saying, "Yes, Chris, tell us about your company – and please tell us about your hair."

Chuck and I both started laughing. Most of the others at our end of the table had not met me before this conference so they didn't understand why we were so amused. When Chuck and I finally stopped giggling and slapping each others' shoulders, I told them my story of going to Istanbul. I also told them Chuck was the very first person who knew me well before my surgery who had seen me in person (not on Zoom) and had the courage to say something about it in front of others. We grabbed the empty tequila bottle and staged a photo to commemorate the moment.

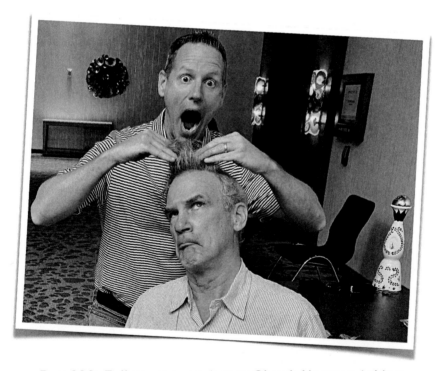

Day 690: Fellow agency owner Chuck Norman taking liberties at Counselors Academy conference in Nashville after we finished the Clase Azul tequila, right.

16. Twenty Years Younger

My two children, Sally and Thomas, were six and eight years old when I gave up on my comb-over and embraced my baldness. They hardly remember me with hair atop my head. They had trouble picturing me with hair when I told them months before going to Istanbul of my plans for surgery. Since then, they've both grown used to me with hair and admit they have trouble remembering me now without hair.

Thomas and his wife Amanda have graced us with two granddaughters, Annie and Eliza. Sally and Alex have recently delivered a grandson, Ansel. A photo of me reading books to Annie is the primary one I save on my iPhone and show people these days who don't believe I used to be bald. A photo of Annie and Eliza taken after Eliza's birth is one I show to compare to often-disbelieving acquaintances. I also love posing with Elena, my step-grandchild, daughter to Catherine and Jorge Villarreal, as she is always smiling, lighting up every photograph with her ample hair.

I recently posted a photo on Facebook of me holding Ansel the day after he was born. It gathered the most likes and comments of any photo I've ever posted on the social media channel. Most of the congratulatory comments focused on Ansel's arrival to earth. Julie Gardner, an early client of my PR firm and a friend who has not seen me in person in years, commented, "Congratulations and you look great, Grandpa Chris!"

I am not a frequent poster on Facebook and am mostly absent on other social media channels other than LinkedIn. My life seems busy enough with managing my small companies, traveling with Jan, visiting my children and grandchildren, organizing close friends for dinner outings, and winding down my life slightly as I've recently turned 65 years old. It might have seemed silly at my age to change my appearance, but I like to think my grandchildren will grow up with their G-Pop's image in their memories and recall me as I remember myself: with hair.

I told Sally and Thomas that my late-age hair follicle surgery might have seemed like a waste of time and money to some people, but I joked that, even if I only lived another year or two, they could say at my funeral, "Well at least Pop lived long enough to see his grandchildren and to see hair return to his head."

Following the pandemic, I don't travel nearly as much as I used to, calling on younger PR firm members to join our digital publishing membership. We've recently pivoted our prospective members based on what the market has delivered to us in the past year. Instead of busy PR firms who are more challenged than ever by their inability to keep staff members aboard to write 100-word stories, we are serving a new group of CEOs who want to be perceived in their market as thought leaders. In the past six months, our largest client is a media owner in Florida who has launched in several markets to expand the brand of their existing political websites.

When I do talk with prospects and tell them I've met all our members in person and would like to fly in to see them, the urgency to do so has been replaced with an acceptance that video calls are adequate substitutions for the effort to travel to their cities

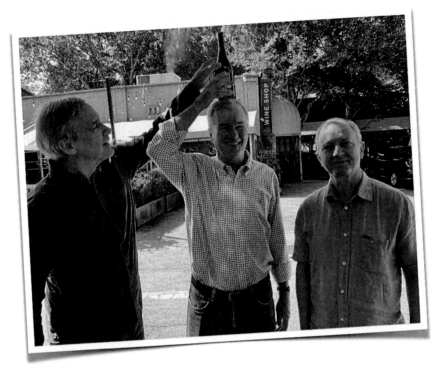

Day 697: Balancing a wine bottle on Mike Egan's head outside Murphy's to update our age 17 photo with Charles Driebe for our quinquennial birthday invitation.

and meet them. Many of them work from home now anyway and don't have offices in which to meet me. So the once-compelling business reasons to change my appearance seemed to have faded with the pandemic and the shifting expansion of our prospective clients.

I'm left to focus on the real reason I made the investment in a "new" head of hair: that it makes me feel better about myself. I was hoping to alleviate a self-perceived obstacle to closing sales – the perception that younger business prospects who once saw me as "old and bald" might think of me now only as "old." Ironically, most acquaintances look at me now and think I look much younger than my age. That never happened when I was bald. Adding more hair to my appearance didn't just eliminate "bald," it impacted both perceptions – if not by others, then at least by me.

I don't walk by mirrors much and I don't gaze at my appearance often, except on Zoom calls. It sounds so vain, but I'm much happier with my appearance participating on Zoom calls with hair than I was the few times I did before the pandemic and before the surgery.

The truth is when I brush my hair in front of a mirror, I am happier with myself. And during most of the day when I work on my computer or work on planting trees, bushes, and flowers on my land at Lake James, I don't see my hair, but I do have a warmer feeling atop my head with hair insulating my previously barren sensitive scalp. I occasionally reach up there and run my fingers through my longer graying hair just to remind myself that it's still there.

Having hair again gives me more confidence about myself. I'm sure some bald people never think twice about their receding hair lines, but in a life blessed with many God-given gifts, it was the one part of myself about which I was insecure. Now, I do feel more content about myself and can worry about shedding my extra few pounds like everybody else.

One other thing that has changed is no one mistakes me for James Taylor or John Malkovich any longer. One day, when my hair was starting to grow out gray and I put on my black glasses and black T-shirt, Jan did tell me I looked like Anderson Cooper. Now that my hair has grown out fully, no one ever says I look like someone else. I just look like me.

When we were young, that generation of hippies talked about "finding ourselves." With hair returning to my head, I feel as if I was once lost and now I've really found myself. I've achieved some of the goals I set for myself in life. Some were probably too ambitious to achieve and I've come to terms with those and realize God had a path for me and I've been extremely lucky to walk it.

When I was in college, I had ambitions to be a great novelist or essayist. I also realized I was neither disciplined nor focused enough to sit down and write a book. It wouldn't surprise me if I was ever diagnosed with a reading or attention-deficit disorder.

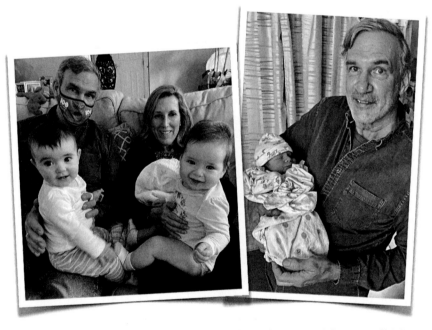

Day 750: My hair arrived in time for photos with grandkids. With granddaughters Eliza, left, Elena, right. Day 884: Welcoming Ansel into the world.

Comprehending large blocks of text was never easy for me. Events that happened to me and my friends – those stories I remember in detail.

Over time, it was telling that I founded a digital publishing company where writing exactly 100-word articles is our brand. That haiku of finishing a perfect 100-word article, telling what would normally be a much longer story in such a few prescribed words, gives me as much joy as finishing my Wordle puzzle each morning. I used to tell myself that I started my career as a newspaper reporter because I knew newspapers would force me to write two or three articles each day and would improve my skills as a writer and that one day, perhaps I would actually turn my attention to writing those novels whose narratives have been marinating in my brain for decades.

One of the reasons my barber Kevin was so excited to take me to Istanbul was he thought if I wrote about our trip in one of my newsletters I'd be able to spread the word about how I changed my appearance and, as he predicted, became so happy with new hair. I went a full year after my surgery before I ventured back into Kevin's barber chair. I don't think Jan could have stood another day. Kevin was so happy to see me and I've been back several times since. Each time, he says, "Chris, you look great! You look 20 years younger!"

On my last trip there, right after he said those exact words, another customer of his walked in and Kevin bragged to him about how he was able to change my appearance by visiting Istanbul. The customer looked confused as my hair looked so natural growing in gray as it has. To convince him I was indeed once bald, I pulled out my photo with Annie, showing the full headscape of baldness from mid 2019. The customer looked at the photo and looked at me and again looked at both. Before taking his seat to wait for Kevin, he said, "Dude, you look 20 years younger!"

Kevin and I laughed and high-fived each other.

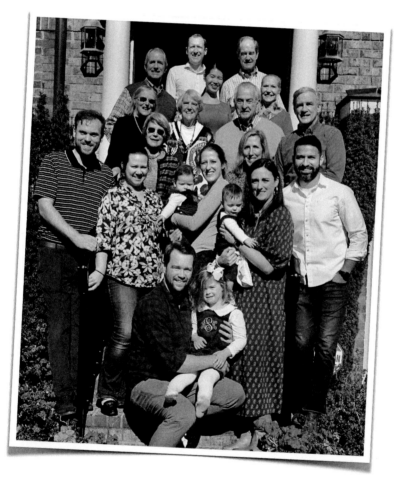

Day 750: My family gathered to celebrate my 65th birthday.

Are there any *good* jokes
about being bald?

We checked … not yet.

What about
Chris Rock's
at the 2022
Oscars?

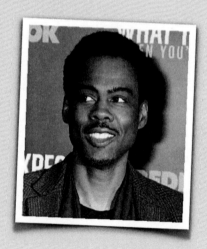

Um … still no.

17. Epilogue: Springtime in Virginia

As I was leaving, Kevin asked again when was I going to write my article about our trip to Istanbul. I assured him I was working on it. I said it was shaping up to be a longer piece and it might be the first article I've ever pitched to a magazine – again one of my personal lifetime goals, along with writing a book. So I began writing this article that I thought would be a few thousand words – too long for my newsletters and, I worried, probably too long to pitch to a magazine. As I launched into telling the story – once having great hair, gradually losing it, having Kevin continually suggest surgery and Jan becoming intrigued by it – the words tumbled out. I'm now approaching 30,000.

The journey of me transplanting hair to the top of my head has not only given me more personal confidence as a salesperson, but it has removed the most insecure part of my self-identity and given me a better image to photograph with my joyful grandchildren. It also turned out to be the key to unlocking my reluctance to sit down and achieve one of my life's main goals – writing a book.

I may have been too scared to do the one thing that I was meant to do, the one I've been avoiding all my life and the one I put off until I was 65 years old. Writing this book about my life with, without, and now again with hair has given me much joy. I don't really care if anyone reads it, though I think opening this subject might be helpful to people who've long worried as I had about their natural baldness.

What I am amazed at today as I type these words is that this journey that began a few years ago in Kevin's barber chair has finally broken the ice on me doing what I have been reluctant to do all my life. In writing this story, I realize I love writing long stories and, in doing so, I have been concurrently feeding the other stories marinating in my head that I may write after finishing this one. That is one outcome of changing my appearance that I never

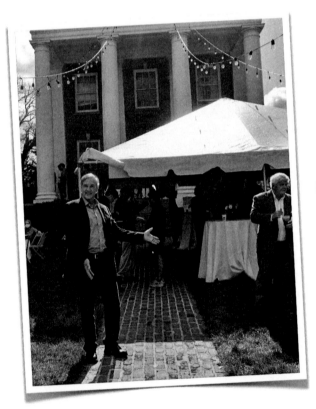

Day 890: Standing on my brick walkway at my delayed 160th UVA fraternity reunion. I built the walkway in August 1977, the week Elvis Presley died.

predicted. Here at my age, I may have finally restarted my life to be the writer I've always wanted to be. May God give me the patience and discipline and time left on this planet to do it – if I was in fact meant to be a book author.

In April 2022, Jan and I flew to Richmond, Virginia to attend that twice-postponed 160th reunion of my fraternity in Charlottesville. As you might expect now, no one at the reunion ever mentioned my new hair. Many of my fraternity brothers congratulated me on recently becoming a grandfather to Ansel and commented on his Facebook post. That and other Facebook photos and the many Zoom calls perhaps pre-conditioned my fraternity brothers and all the others in my life to already have grown used to me with what buddy Dr. TC now calls my "new gray mane."

The surprises I had envisioned for year 2020 didn't work out the way I had planned. Yet, many other positive things have happened along the way and I'm so very glad I went to Istanbul. I may return one day and finish filling in the bald spot on the back of my head with hairs from under my chin that reside there now to grow a beard.

While we were in Richmond, Jan and I met a couple for lunch on a cafe patio. The couple decades ago lived down the street from Jan and her first husband. We had met once years ago for a quick drink in a Richmond bar. Of course, they didn't remember me that well and, when we sat outside in the beautiful Richmond spring weather, they mostly caught up with Jan and stories about their old friends as I listened and occasionally commented.

Jan sat across from me at our table and was looking at me a bit more often than usual. Jan and I love each other and we enjoy doing so many activities together that we have in common, but we, like many married couples, don't compliment each other as much as perhaps we should. I don't believe we feel a deficit in that area, but when we do take the time to make such comments, I'm sure she appreciates it as much as do I.

Walking to the car from the cafe, Jan said something out of character, out of the blue.

"I was looking at you across the table," she said. "I was thinking how handsome you look."

It was a simple comment, but one I hadn't heard often from Jan and certainly not in that matter-of-fact tone conveying to me that she really meant it. Maybe now that she felt free to express that she thought I was handsome, I really could feel complete as a man. I wondered if that $7,000 investment in my surgery was worth just this one moment to hear her say that phrase so casually and sincerely. It caused me to tear up and to be thankful that she had encouraged me to change my headscape more than two years earlier and that she was as pleased with the outcome as I was.

I thought, given all that we had been through since we met when I was a determined yet still insecure entrepreneur, that it didn't really matter if no one else ever again mentions my hair or says I look younger. What mattered at that moment was that we were happy with each other and happy with ourselves and with all the blessings God has given us.

And truly, in life, is there a more important achievement one can attain?

– The End –

*For more on Headscape and hair transplantation,
visit www.headscape.me*

Photography credits:

Page 2: J. Spalding Schroder, M.D.

Page 6: The Westminster Schools, Lynx, 1969, 1970

Page 7: J. Spalding Schroder, M.D.

Page 8: James "Jim" Russell

Page 10: U.S. Government official photos

Page 12: J. Spalding Schroder, M.D.

Page 12: Rickey Pittman, *The Augusta Chronicle*

Page 13, 131: Schroder Family photos

Page 15: Callender Patterson

Page 16: Lars Matré

Page 21: Designed by Chris Schroder

Page 24: Dilbert, Scott Adams, Andrews McMeel Syndication

Page 29: David Glueck, *Daily Report*

Page 31: Dreamstime.com: © Laurence Agron

Page 31: The Rock photo: © Starstock

Page 34: Gabrielle Ward Whalen

Page 37: Jae Robbins, Jessica Childers, Resource Branding

Page 40: Tom Murphy; Jack Hollingsworth

Page 43: Jan Schroder

Page 44: David Hinton for Oxford Center; Greg Harding Films

Page 50: Selfie by Chris Schroder, group shot by table-mates

Page 57: Michael Schroder

Page 61, 62: Chris Schroder

Page 65: Tolga Sari for Estefirst

Page 67: Tolga Sari for Estefirst
Page 68: Chris Schroder; Kevin Serani
Page 70: Chris Schroder
Page 73: Michael Schroder
Page 74: Kevin Serani
Page 78: Gökhan Er, Arista Communications
Page 84, 85, 88: Chris Schroder
Page 86: Jan Schroder
Page 90: Murphy's wait staff
Page 93: J. Spalding Schroder, M.D.
Page 94: Chris Schroder
Page 97: Jan Schroder
Page 98-104: Chris Schroder
Page 106: Dreamstime: © Kysa
Page 109, 110, 116: Chris Schroder
Page 112: Jan Schroder
Page 113: Jean Rollins
Page 119: Jan Schroder; Thomas Schroder
Page 120: Chris Schroder
Page 123: Richelle Brooks for Schroder PR
Page 127: Murphy's Wait Staff
Page 128: Catherine Villarreal
Page 128: Alex Fritz
Page 132: Dreamstime.com: © Laurence Agron
Page 134: Maddie Robinson Photography
Page 141: Greg Harding Films

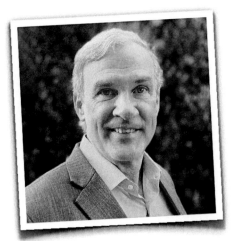

About the Author

Chris Schroder worked for six daily newspapers, serving first as a reporter, then editor, promotions director, creative director and advertising director – winning awards in several states for his reporting and print advertisement design.

He started and served as publisher of his Atlanta neighborhood newspapers in 1994, selling them to real estate developer Tom Cousins in 2000. He then built a PR firm, selling it to The Wilbert Group in November 2017. He's the creator and producer of the Moments video series on SaportaReport.com, where he was founding member and publisher. He developed and continues to publish dozens of newsletters and websites across the USA with his digital publishing firm, The 100 Companies.

Chris is a graduate of the University of Virginia, where he majored in English and was executive editor of *The Declaration*. He spends his spare time with friends, listening to music, hiking, biking and golfing – and his favorite activity – visiting with wife Jan their four children, three granddaughters and one grandson.